What's Shakin'

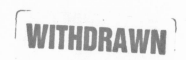

What's Shakin'

✦

An Insider's Look at the Humorous Side of Parkinson's Disease

John Brissette
FOREWORD
BY TOM RADEMACHER
COLUMNIST, GRAND RAPIDS
PRESS

iUniverse, Inc.
New York Lincoln Shanghai

What's Shakin'
An Insider's Look at the Humorous Side of Parkinson's Disease

Copyright © 2007 by John Brissette

iUniverse books may be ordered through booksellers or by contacting:

iUniverse
2021 Pine Lake Road, Suite 100
Lincoln, NE 68512
www.iuniverse.com
1-800-Authors (1-800-288-4677)

ISBN: 978-0-595-42500-6 (pbk)
ISBN: 978-0-595-88549-7 (cloth)

Printed in the United States of America

This book is dedicated to my dearest family and friends who have made my life much easier to handle and have given me a reason to go on.

To:

My wife Kathy; who has had to bear the burden of my disease. She has been by my side every step of the way, and has endured more sorrow and sacrifice than anyone should have to. I could not have made it without you. I love you dearly.

My mom and dad; who have always been there for me through the good times and the bad, the happy and the sad, and whose love has shown me that I will never be alone.

My daughter Elizabeth and my son Jason; whom I love dearly and am so proud of. From the first day that you came into my life you have brought me joy and happiness. I regret that I will not be here by your side as long as I wanted to, but I hope I will be in your memory forever.

My sister Barbara and her family; whose love, support and the special times we share mean a great deal to me. Our love and bond has grown with each passing year.

My best friends Patrick and Jim; who I couldn't imagine being any closer to than if we were brothers. Thanks for the good times, thanks for your love and your support. Thanks for your friendship.

Kathy's mom; who has always treated me as if I were her own. Thank you. Her brother Steve and his family, your love and friendship I cherish.

My dog Tyler; who is a friend bar-none. He is the greatest dog I have ever known. Even on my worst days he has brought a smile to my face. From the first day I brought you home you have shown a sweetness and gentleness that is unsurpassed.

A special thanks to God; who gave me the ability to laugh at myself, take what life doles out to me and make the best of it. I have been able to find joy and laughter in every dark cloud and know tomorrow will be a sunnier day.

Acknowledgements

A special thanks to:
Cover Photo by James Prisby, Hudsonville, MI
Illustrations by Don Dooley, A very talented young artist Rockford, MI

Contents

FOREWORD

By
Tom Rademacher
Columnist, The Grand Rapids Press

One of the best self-help books you might ever own? You're holding it in your hands.

John Brissette didn't set out to write something for your soul, but in his own humble and self-deprecating way, he provides the rest of us something of a road map by which we might chart a better course for lives too often steeped in apathy and self-absorption.

Where else, after all, have you ever come across a subtitle like "An Insider's Look at the Humorous Side of Parkinson's Disease?"

The first time I ever laid eyes on John Brissette, he was wildly waving his arms in the air while reveling listeners with a tale of how, after decades of unsuccessful deer-hunting, he'd finally bagged his first whitetail. But instead of extolling the merits of his hunting prowess, he was marveling at how he was able to dispatch a wild animal despite all the mistakes he'd committed. He had a little audience eating out of his hand, and I thought to myself, "This guy's some storyteller."

That suspicion would manifest itself many times over as I read the manuscript that would become this book. And I can guarantee that, like me, you'll laugh out loud at the capers John Brissette has accidentally manufactured and endured while dealing with a debilitating disease like Parkinson's.

Here's a guy who's been decked by a runaway golf cart, fallen flat on the concrete floor of a big-box store, and suffered the indignity of filling his shoes with urine in front of a bunch of gawking teen-agers. In his effort to perform some home repairs to his sister's home, he managed to nearly destroy a bathroom, spilled a gallon of paint onto expensive carpet, put a hole in their wall, and severed a gas line with a hedge trimmer. In the process, he caused more than $320 in damages.

Another person might have checked out. John Brissette, who lives with the realization that his disease gets worse, just laughs.

I've made a living nearly 30 years as a newspaperman, and in writing articles and columns about thousands of people facing life on life's terms, I've rarely met a gem like John Brissette.

He'll tell you in the final chapter of this book, appropriately entitled "Eureka," how he's discovered the secret of getting up every day, even with Parkinson's. It's rooted in the realization that even the best-laid plans can be obliterated when criss-crossed by fate or bad luck or karma or whatever you want to call it.

John Brissette maintains that you've got two choices when faced with a calamity: Either wallow in grief, or get on with it.

"Wasting precious time trying to understand why bad things happen to us gets us nowhere," he writes. "Eventually, it will introduce us to the paths of self-pity and depression. Choose the other path."

It takes a generous person to embrace pathos, and consider the bittersweet gifts it sometimes has to offer. John Brissette is up to the task, extending his trembling reach with a smile.

1

THE BOMB

THE BOMB

"John, I believe you have Parkinson's disease," Dr. Neuman said with a compassionate look in his eyes.

I was speechless. It was a left hook out of nowhere. I couldn't have Parkinson's. I didn't know much about the disease, but I did know it was an old persons disease (or so I thought). I was only 45. This couldn't be. I was stunned and confused. I wasn't at all prepared for this. My mind was racing through a jumbled network of incoherent thoughts. Sifting through a multitude of mixed emotions I tried to bring myself back to reality.

My head filled with questions and I began to spit them out one after the other. For twenty minutes Dr. Neuman sat and patiently answered all my questions: "Is it life threatening?" "No, but it will affect the quality of your life". "What are the symptoms?" "Tremors in the hand, head, and legs, rigidity in the muscles effecting walk, speech, and motor skills". "Is there a cure?" "No, there is no cure. It is a degenerative disease, but there are numerous drugs available that work very well in controlling the symptoms, and there is some hope that a cure will be found soon," and so on.

When we were finished, Dr. Neuman rose, held out his hand, and said he wished he had better news. He said if I had any further questions to please feel free to call him at any time. With that he handed me some literature on Parkinson's disease, and explained to me that there were several support groups available for Parkinson's patients if I desired one. Inside I was furious. I didn't need any damn support group! Hell, I wasn't convinced I even had Parkinson's.

As I left his office and wandered down the hall, I entered the "OZONE." You know that state of mind, where everything is going on around you but you are not really a part of it; you are one step out of sync, like another world is going on all around you. I found my car, slid into my seat, and sat there for twenty minutes.

The ride home was a unique one. I didn't turn on the radio, I didn't put in a CD, I didn't say a word, oh God, how that was going to change. What was I going to tell my wife, Kathy? How was this going to affect our marriage? How was this going to affect my work? How were my mom and dad going to handle this? How were my children going to handle this? The questions kept coming and coming and I had no answers! But first, I had to tell Kathy. This was definitely going to affect her life.

This was a second marriage for both of us. We were very happy. She was not merely the girl I loved; she was also one of my best friends. We had an age difference of ten years. In spite of what some people might say this is really a lot, especially the older you get. When you can't do the physical things like you used to it can be a burden to any relationship. When you throw Parkinson's into the mix it can be a major detriment to any marriage, no matter how strong. When I thought about the problems that Parkinson's would bring, I felt like an old man before his time. A man that couldn't care for himself. A man that couldn't provide for his family. A useless man. Those were the concerns that began to occupy my mind.

I pulled into my driveway and parked the car. I started to open the door and a feeling of nausea enveloped me. I vomited. I prayed Kathy wasn't watching. I wiped my mouth and sat there for a few moments. It seemed like I had been gone an eternity. As I gripped the door handle I noticed my hand was visibly shaking. I opened the car door, got out, and walked up to the front porch. I was somewhat startled as Kathy opened the front door and greeted me with a big hug and asked, "What did the doctor say?" As I looked into her eyes I could see her expression change. "What's wrong?" she uttered. At that very moment I decided to tell her everything.

"Kathy, wait a minute, OK?" I walked past her and went into the kitchen for a beer. "What's wrong?" I could hear the fear in her voice. I didn't answer her. I popped the top on a cold one and guzzled half of it down in one long gulp. I walked back into the living room, sat next to her, and placed her hand in my lap. I repeated everything that Dr. Neuman had told me. I emphasized three things ... That Parkinson's was a degenerative disease, there was no cure, but there were drugs available that did a very good job of controlling the symptoms.

When we were finished, tears were running down her cheek. I hated myself for hurting her. We embraced in silence. Thus began my life with Parkinson's. My life would never be the same.

As I stated before, as far as I knew Parkinson's was an old person's disease. I was only 45—how could this be? It was unacceptable. Just because one doctor said I had Parkinson's didn't mean it was true. So, I went back to my family physician Dr. Baer, who is an outstanding young doctor, and the first to suspect the tremor might be more than just nerve damage. I asked him for a referral and made an appointment. This doctor confirmed the diagnosis ... I had Parkinson's disease. For the second time in less than a week I was devastated.

Over the next couple of weeks I found myself becoming short tempered, uneasy and sometimes just down right ornery. I kept asking myself, "Why did this happen to me? What did I ever do to deserve this? I'm not a bad person, why me?" I wish I had the answers but I couldn't come up with any. I wanted them. I needed them.

It had been a couple of weeks since I learned of my Parkinson's and as yet, I still hadn't told my parents. (I come from a very close family and I was worried about the effect this was going to have on them). The greatest gift my mom and dad have ever given me is that no matter what the circumstances were they have always been there for me. They have shared my joys and my sorrows, my laughter and my tears, and through it all they have been by my side every step of the way.

I was thankful for the 3-hour drive to Royal Oak because it gave me an opportunity to rehearse what I was going to say. Unfortunately, nothing could prepare me for what I had to do. I had called my mom and dad the day before and told them that I would be stopping by around noon to discuss something with them.

When I arrived, my mom was in the kitchen preparing lunch. As always, she wasn't just making bologna sandwiches, she had gone out of her way to make chicken salad (one of my favorites), homemade rolls, and sliced cantaloupe. But that's the way she has always been. My mom never puts herself first; she has always been concerned about everyone else's needs before her own.

I told my parents that we would talk after we ate. They said that would be fine, but I could see the concerned look on their faces ... they knew something was wrong. After lunch we went into the living room and I unfolded my story. As I was talking, I could see the tears building in their eyes. When I was finished I looked at them and could immediately read their expressions. The look on their faces must have been similar to the look on my face when Dr. Neuman told me I had Parkinson's ... except there was something different, it was more intense. But I knew that look too.

When my son Jason was five he was injured very seriously in a car accident. The neuro-surgeon came down and said, "If your son makes it through the night ..." I did not hear another word after that. My God, how can you tell a parent that? The terror of that statement, the terror of what it meant, was unbearable. There is no sorrow, no devastation, and no emptiness like a parent feels when dealing with the loss of a child. That was the look I now saw on my mom and dads face. (In case you are wondering, my son made it through the night, and is just fine now.)

As we gazed into each other's eyes, I struggled to fight back my tears. My dad said quietly, "You know John, anything we can do for you, anything you need, anything at all, all you have to do is ask". I gave my dad a simple nod. I sank into my mother's arms, she held me close, and I wept.

Over the next few weeks the bomb had been dropped on everyone, including my two children, Jason and Beth, who were devastated with the news. They had faced two major tragedies in their young lives: the divorce of their parents and now my illness. I hurt deeply for them.

I also had to tell my two best friends, Pat (who I have known my whole life) and Jim (who I have known since college). Although they seemed to accept the news, I'm sure they were wondering how this was going to affect our friendship.

It was an emotional and difficult time for everyone but I was glad it was over. It felt like a great weight had been lifted off my shoulders. I could now concentrate my concerns and efforts on all the other things yet to come.

THE DISEASE

One of the frustrating things about Parkinson's disease is determining what medication to use. What works well for one patient may not work well for another. What works well today may not work well tomorrow. What dosage was ample yesterday is not enough for today. In addition, the doctor and patient must also grapple with the never-ending battle of weighing the medication's side effects versus the Parkinson's symptoms. Many have told me that the cure for Parkinson's is just over the horizon. This is wonderful news to all who are stricken with Parkinson's disease, but until that day becomes a reality, we must deal with the problems, as they exist.

In spite of the side effects, I find these medications a gift from God. I often think of how miserable life must have been for all previous Parkinson's patients who did not have these wonder drugs available to them. It must have been pure hell.

Parkinson's is not only a debilitating disease; it is a humiliating and demeaning disease. It takes a normal, healthy, and confident individual and turns him into an object of stares, disgust, and diminishes the ability to care for himself. It is terrifying to think what one would have to endure without family and friends to help them along the way.

Parkinson's disease occurs when certain cells in the brain that produce a chemical called Dopamine malfunction or die. Dopamine is a neuro-transmitter, which enables signals to and from the brain to be transmitted quickly and smoothly. When the first symptom of Parkinson's disease shows itself, 80% of the dopamine-producing cells are already either malfunctioning or dead. Parkinson's is a degenerative disease and as yet there is no cure.

I have had Parkinson's for ten years. During this time I have displayed most of the of the disease's symptoms as well as most of the side effects of the medications. Following is a list including both symptoms and side effects and the general chronological order in which they occurred. Also noted (in bold face type) are some humorous stories included in this book. All the stories are true, though a few have been embellished a little to further your enjoyment and to protect the innocent. I hope you find them amusing.

After reading this book, if I can leave you with anything, I would like it be these two thoughts 1) The ability to laugh at one's self is precious; and 2) When you look up in the sky, look beyond the gray clouds and see the glorious sun drenched blue skies above.

SYMPTOMS (D) AND SIDE EFFECTS (S)

Tremors (D): **THE SPEECH**

Rigidity (D): **THE CALL**

Grip (D): **THE BALL WASHER**

Shuffled walk (D): **THE SHOES**

Drowsiness (S): **THE DRIVE**

Balance (D): **THE SEWER DISPLAY**
THE JUNKYARD
GREEN KNEES AND TP

Slurred Speech (D

Confusion (S): **THE GOLF CART**

Insomnia(S)

Personality Changes(S)

Constipation(S): **THE CONTEST**

Difficulty swallowing (D)

Shortness of breath (D)

Hallucinations (S) **THE WOMEN**
               THE NIGHT VISITORS

Combination of symptoms (D & S) **NO PARKING**
                             LET IT RIDE
                             THE HANDYMAN

2

THE SPEECH

THE SPEECH

TREMORS

This is where it all began. While sitting at my office desk one day, I noticed a tremor in my little finger. It never subsided. Originally it was misdiagnosed as nerve damage, but upon further testing it was later diagnosed as Parkinson's disease. After this initial tremor made itself known the disease attacked all my fingers, my left hand, my left arm, my right side and so on. All Parkinson's patients are victimized by the "shakes" or "The Whips and Jingles" as my father-in-law called it. The following story; "The Speech", is a humorous event involving the shakes.

I was forced to retire (due to Parkinson's) two years ago, as the General Manager of a Grand Rapids, MI, hotel. My boss, Tim Garner, who had been with me from my early diagnosis of Parkinson's until my retirement, was the greatest boss I ever had. He was dedicated to his job, and I never saw him give less than 100%. He was understanding and truly cared about his employees. During my ten-year battle with Parkinson's, Tim never once made me feel like my job was in jeopardy and supported me at every turn. I admired him greatly. That is why, when I was asked to give a speech at our annual management meeting, in his honor, I said "yes" without thought or hesitation.

Our company had two divisions: a hotel side, and a golf course side. For the first time, the golf division staff (who we never really had contact with) was also going to be included in our meeting as a tribute to Tim. I was informed that I was going to be one of four people paying a verbal tribute to him.

Now, you may think that, being a hotel General Manager who meets hundreds of different people every day, I would be a gregarious soul. WRONG. Nothing could be further from the truth. I am an ordained introvert. Volunteering to give a speech, in a banquet room full of people, was something I wouldn't do being of sound mind and body.

Everyday following my acceptance I did a ritualistic butt kicking and asked myself how I could have ever agreed to give "the speech". To make matters worse, not only were the managers of the golf division going to be in attendance, but also all the corporate office staff.

The day we left for Cincinnati (where our home office was) I was a mess. I had cramps, a headache, an upset stomach, and had to stop the car every 40 minutes for a potty break. I had no dinner that night or breakfast in the morning. My nerves were shot. I was frazzled. I felt like passing out. As the meeting began the next morning, to my horror I found out that I was going to be the last speaker. My God, I didn't want to be last—I wanted this over.

I had told my good friend Bob Kolomak, General Manager of the Hampton Inn in Saginaw, MI, what I was going through. He continually tried to ease my anxiety, but to no avail. As Mr. Garner was called up to the front of the room I noticed my sweaty hands ... they were shaking OH NO ... PLEASE NOT NOW ... DID I FORGET? ... Yes—In my frenzied state I forgot to take my medicine. I quickly gobbled down a couple of pills; would they work on time? Would it be enough? Would I be frozen in my chair? What was I going to do?

The third speaker was just closing and I swear I thought I was going to fill my pants. Then I could hear the introduction begin and the words, "Our general manager from Grand Rapids, John Brissette." Then applause.

Feet don't fail me now.... I rose to my feet and started to walk. I was a little rigid but I *was* walking. With "the speech" in hand I moved precariously up to the podium, stood behind the mike, and froze. The only thing that was moving were my arms and hands ... wildly, not just from my nerves, but from the Parkinson's "shimmy" too.

I just stood there in front of everyone, my hands shaking uncontrollably. Then I made a huge mistake. Have you ever had that little man in your head tell you not to do something and regretfully you shove him aside and do it anyway? That's what happened to me. I could hear myself say, "Don't do it you idiot." As I passed "the speech" from one hand to the other, all I was able to do was shred it into a million pieces, in front of everyone. I looked out into the audience and could read their faces. Those who knew me stared at me with hurt and pity; those who didn't know me stared with fear and confusion. I felt like crying. This was pure hell.

I don't know what happened next. I can't explain it—it was a miracle—let's call it divine intervention.

My physical contortions were stopping because the drugs were taking effect. I was breathing easier. I was calming down. I knew I was going to be all right. Then it happened, like when you relentlessly try to remember something but can't. Out of nowhere ... WHAMO! It comes to you. My head filled with one thought: I turned to Mr. Garner and said, "Ya know Tim, when you hired me, you said you were looking for a mover and a shaker ... well, I'm not a very good mover, but I'm one hell of a shaker."

The audience erupted in a deafening roar of laughter, stood up, and gave me a continuous standing ovation. End of speech, they were mine.

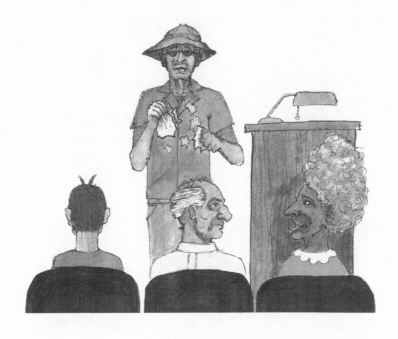

3

THE CALL

THE CALL

RIGIDITY

Another symptom of Parkinson's disease is rigidity. Rigidity is the stiffening of the muscles that prohibits the patient from moving freely. In its severest state, it is called "freezing", where the patient is unable to move at all. Freezing can occur while standing, walking, or in the prone position. It is particularly common for me to be walking in full stride and suddenly come to a complete stop, unable to move. It requires my total concentration or someone to push me gently in order to start moving again. My wife is so tuned in to this, sometimes she pushes me when I'm just standing there thinking.

The following is a humorous look at rigidity.

Because I have difficulty sleeping some nights, I often sleep downstairs on my recliner. This enables my wife to get an undisturbed night's sleep. On one such evening I awoke at 2:30 A.M. and quickly determined I was unable to move. I was "frozen" in my recliner and was only able to move my arms. Drowsy and confused I began to feel very uneasy. I needed to wake Kathy but how would I do it? I wasn't sure she could hear me from upstairs.

Then a great idea hit me. As the general manager of a hotel, I have staff on duty 24 hours a day. So I called my night auditor (I always keep a phone at my side) and asked her to call my house. I told her to let the phone ring until my wife answered and then tell her that I was frozen downstairs and needed her help. I hung up the phone and waited. In a few moments the phone rang. It rang and rang, but my wife did not answer. I then remembered I had taken the phone out of our bedroom earlier in the day and had forgotten to return it.

As I became more uneasy, I decided that I might be able to wake Kathy if I yelled loud enough. So I took a deep breath and yelled as loud as I could "Kathy!" over and over again. I yelled for about two minutes, but failed to get any response.

Then another idea hit me. Perhaps I could wake our dog Tyler who sleeps in our bedroom (usually in our bed). If I could rouse him, maybe he would scratch at the door and wake Kathy (after all, dogs were supposed to have great hearing, weren't they?). I called Tyler for several minutes … no response. He remained oblivious to my predicament. Either he didn't hear me or he was ignoring me because it gave him more room in our bed (which was more likely the case). Either way, I still had a problem.

I was beginning to become quite panicky. Now I had to go to the bathroom too. Although I was only in my under shorts and t-shirt I was beginning to sweat quite badly. I was breathing rapidly and the urge to go potty was increasing. Unable to calm myself down, I thought my only other option was to call my neighbor Bill Dick. I dialed his number. It rang once, and I quickly hung up. My God it was 2:30 A.M., what was I going to say? I frantically searched for another option. One kept coming up but I kept pushing it away … I didn't want to do that. Finally, with no other solution in sight, I called 9-1-1

"Hello—this is 9-1-1 emergency, how can I help you?" "This is John Brissette, I live at 111 Melody Lane, I have Parkinson's disease and I'm frozen in my recliner and I can't move."

"One moment Mr. Brissette," and she put me on hold. After what seemed like an eternity the operator finally came on again and said, "Did you pay your bill?"

"What? What in the heck are you talking about? Pay what bill?" "Your heating bill, you said you were cold."

"NO, I said I am frozen. To a Parkinson's patient that means we are unable to move. "Ma'am, let me start again—what I need is a police officer to come to my house, ring the doorbell and wake up my wife so she can assist me. I'm unable to move at all because of my Parkinson's and I am starting to cramp up. Please tell the officer not to come over with his siren blaring and his lights flashing as it will scare my wife and disturb my neighbors. OK?" She said, "OK"

I hung up the phone and waited. In about five minutes I could hear the police siren blaring before I saw red and blue lights flashing. Then there came a banging at the door and all hell broke loose. Tyler began barking uncontrollably and I could hear my wife screaming, "What's going on, oh my God the police, what's going on?" So I started screaming, "Kathy it's ok, I called the police. I'm frozen in my chair," over and over again. The police kept ringing our doorbell, the dog kept barking and the lights kept flashing.

My wife frantically came downstairs and opened the front door. The police officer stated that I had called 9-1-1 and was having a problem. He asked if he could come in and speak to me. Kathy said "OK". The police officer came in to our den, where I was laying in my underwear and asked me what my problem was. I said that I was a Parkinson's patient and I was frozen in my chair. He looked at me with a confused expression on his face and said, "Why don't you cover up with a blanket?"

OH LORD, HERE WE GO AGAIN

4

THE SHOES

THE SHOES

SLOWNESS OF MOVEMENT/SHUFFLED WALK

At this point in my life I was experiencing a new symptom of Parkinson's disease, the shuffled gait. All I needed was a white wig and to say 'SHEEES GOOONE" and I would have made a perfect double for Tim Conway's character the "old man." When I was on my medication I moved normally, but without it my stride (and I use that word very loosely) was only a couple of inches. If we were to run the 100-yard dash, you could spot me 98 yards and still win. My feet, especially my toes, became very sensitive. When I shuffle along, I ram my tender tootsies into the toes of my shoes over and over again. After awhile they become unbearably sore.

I love the game of golf, but it has never really loved me. I am continually trying to improve my game by one means or another. I have played every golf ball imaginable, purchased numerous putters, bought oodles of gimmicks, training aids and even voodoo incantations, but nothing has really worked. One summer, I was in the need of a new pair of golf shoes; after all, mine were almost a year old. So I decided to order a new pair of shoes through my boss, Mr. Garner, who also supervised the golf division of our company. I was a little reluctant (I've never bought shoes without trying them on first), but he assured me that everything would be alright. So I gave him my shoe size, and my money, and the shoes were ordered.

When the package arrived from UPS, I wasted no time. I tore open the box and pulled out my new golf shoes. They were beautiful. They were white saddle shoes, trimmed with black and brown-tooled leather. They retailed at most sporting good stores for $149. Due to the discount I only paid $89. These were the finest and most expensive shoes I had ever purchased. I put them on immediately. Hmm, a little snug I thought ... but weren't all new shoes a little snug—until they got broken in, that is? I couldn't wait to try them out.

It had been a rainy Friday morning, but the rain had stopped now. The sky was overcast but it was 79 degrees and it looked like it might clear up. I wanted to wear my new shoes and hit a few, so I called Kathy and asked her if she wanted to play golf after work. She said she didn't want to play, but she would ride along with me if it wasn't raining.

I phoned one of the golf courses we play, and to my disappointment was informed that they had a golf outing that morning and early afternoon. We would be able to get out after 3:00 P.M. Not what I had hoped for, but I wanted to play so I made a tee time.

There was no mistaking it—my new golf shoes were a little snug. I decided to take this opportunity to try and stretch them a little by wearing them the rest of the afternoon. I do not have many faults, but one of the few I do have is that I can be bull-headed. These shoes were going to be just fine, I told myself.

After Kathy had returned home she asked me several times, "How do you like your shoes?" To which I quickly responded (sorry to steal your line Tony), "They're GREAT." The truth was, they were killing me, but I'll be damned if I was going to take my shoes off. Besides, all they needed was a little stretching, right?

Well, it was finally time to head over to the golf course. "Aren't you going to change your shoes?" Kathy asked as we climbed into the car. "No, I'll just wear them over there, no point in changing." The real reason was my feet were so sore and swollen, if I took them off, I didn't think I could get my feet back into them again.

When we arrived at the course, we could see that the golf outing was still going on, and it looked like it would continue for some time. Everyone had finished their round of golf, but they were still partying around the clubhouse. I went into the pro shop and was told that we could go right out.

As I walked up to the first tee Kathy said, "What's wrong?" "What do you mean?" I replied. Kathy said, "You are walking kind of funny." "Oh, I guess my shoes are a little stiff." I drove the ball and we took off. Well let me tell you, I was miserable. I thought my toes were going to fall off. We finished #1 and went on to the next hole. When I walked over to the #2 tee, my step changed to a shuffle. A new and intense pain struck my feet. Those poor little appendages were being rammed into the ends of my shoes with every step.

Kathy commented, "You look like you are in real pain, let's go home."

"No I'll be alright, my shoes just need a little breaking in. That's all." I hobbled up to the tee box and drove the ball.

The #2 green is on a good size hill. I hit my second shot through the green and down the side of the hill. When I got to the green, I grabbed my sand wedge and my putter and shuffled off to the far side of the green. I took two steps down the hill, let out an audible moan, twirled and went back up to the edge of the green. I bent over in excruciating pain. All I could think about was how I was ever going to finish this round. WHAT A DOPE.

Then a brilliant idea struck me. OH, OH—There was no way I could walk down any of these hills forward so—BADA BOOM—I would just walk down the hills backwards. DOUBLE DOPE.

I told Kathy to pick up my ball. She did, shook her head, and mumbled something about going home. I gave myself a bogey and walked over to the next tee.

The third hole has three interesting facets: 1) The green is on a very large hill; 2) It has trees and a pond 2/3 of the way around the green; 3) It backs up to the clubhouse. Arriving at the third tee, we could hear the people from the golf outing hooting and hollering, obviously having a very good time.

I hit a beautiful drive right down the center of the fairway about 240 yards. I always liked this hole. If you play it well you can show off to the people who are sitting outside the clubhouse watching you hit up. I drove up to my ball and got out of the cart. It was 173 yards to the center of the green. I wanted to hit a great shot. I pulled out my 4-iron, addressed the ball ("helloooooo baaall", for all of you Honeymooner fans), and smacked a beautiful shot that landed on the green, bounced twice, and rolled off the back edge.

I drove the cart up to the front of the green (the hill was too steep to drive on), got out, and shuffled across the green to look for my ball. I stood on top of the hill and looked down. I could see that my ball had come to rest at the bottom of the hill about ten feet from the pond. I was disappointed because I had hit a really good shot, and with the green being soft from all that rain it should have held.

I stood there deciding how to hit my next shot and trying to figure out if there was any other way to get to my ball without going down that damn hill. There was not. I was going to have to go down backwards—*Please God help me … Let me see the light.*

The one good thing about this green was that the top half of the hill had a lot of trees on it, and probably no one could see me. I took my sand wedge, stopped at the edge of the green, turned around and took a deep breath. After saying a little prayer I took my first step backward down the hill. Under normal circumstances performing this maneuver should have been relatively easy. However, with Parkinson's and feet that felt like I had just walked barefoot through a cactus farm ... "what in the hell was I thinking?"

About the fourth step backwards I caught my heel on a root. I don't know which came first, the lunge backwards or the scream, but that's what started things rolling (no pun intended). At first, the scream was a shrill shriek (try and say that 3 times) but then it turned into an ooooo-hhhaaaaahh, oooooohhhhhaaaaahhhh, aaaaaaaaahhhhhhhhhh. I was now doing a goose step backwards with HUGE steps trying not to fall. My feet felt like I had poured tacks in my socks. My strides were getting longer, almost uncontrollable. My arms were flailing as if hornets were attacking me. Every part of my body was moving in a different direction trying to gain balance.

Alas, it was not going to happen. With 65 pairs of red-liquored eyes fixed on me from the clubhouse, I performed a magnificent backwards one-and-a half gainer in the tuck position.

S P L A S H! I know it wasn't a 9.9 but it sure deserved at least a 9.6.

The guffaws and belly laughs from the clubhouse were unmistakable and not appreciated.

When my head popped up out of the water all I could see was Kathy standing at the top of the hill, bent over, and shaking uncontrollably. She might have been crying ... but I don't think so.

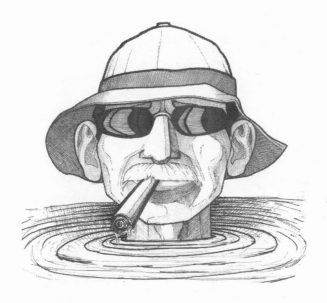

5

GETTING OVER THE HUMP

GETTING OVER THE HUMP

During the first eight years of my treatment, I had always insisted on minimum strengths and dosages of my medications, because the side effects of these drugs were so numerous and severe. However, in the last few years my body's demand for dopamine has increased drastically and as a result the most important thing for me has become what I call "getting over the hump."

As I previously stated, Parkinson's is a degenerative disease. When you see the first symptoms of Parkinson's, 80% of the cells that produce a substance called dopamine are either malfunctioning or dead. Dopamine is a neuro-transmitter that enables signals to and from the brain to move quickly and smoothly. When dopamine is lacking, movements by the individual are jerky or slow.

The doctor and patient face a constant challenge in determining what type of medication and what dosage will best control the symptoms. The ironic thing is that a drug that is unacceptable now may be more than acceptable in the future. Because of the many different medications available, experimentation of what might work best for a patient is common.

When my medication is "on" and everything is hunky dory it's hard for anyone to tell that there is anything wrong with me. Sometimes it's even hard for me to tell. I move, act, and talk normally. This is fantastic. This is the way I want to be, however, this can be a problem. "How can this be a problem?" you ask. The problem is that I am so close to normal I often forget to take my medications.

This wasn't a real problem in my early stages of Parkinson's. My symptoms were not that pronounced or severe, so most of the time I merely had to take my next dosage of medicine to maintain normalcy. But today it is no longer that easy. Taking one more pill no longer does it for me. As a result the daily conflict I face is "What will it take to get me over the hump," and additionally, how do I maintain it. Some days I fail to make it at all.

The challenge is this … if I don't take enough medicine and fail to get over the hump I am really uncomfortable. I can move my feet only a few inches at a time, if I can move them at all. I can barely use my hands. I cannot swallow easily, my breathing is shallow, I drool, and I shake uncontrollably. I am a mess. If I am not trying to move, my outward appearance seems to be somewhat normal. However, on the inside I am panicky, in distress and miserable. Others can understand me when I converse and I am very easy to deal with, so people are comfortable being around me. I am not an object of anyone's attention.

If I over medicate, though, my body's metabolism speeds up tenfold. I cannot sit still. I have to be doing something. My speech is severely slurred and soft. I am extremely difficult to understand. The ironic thing is that I have the *uncontrollable urge to talk*. I cannot stop. (I have to talk to someone even if it's to myself and that's what I usually do).

I am difficult to be around. I also believe that I can do things that I am just not capable of doing and usually get myself into trouble. I am a totally different person. I am uncontrollable. I act and look goofy. More times than I care to remember I have brought my wife and my mother to tears because they long for me to be back the way I was before. When I'm in this state it hurts me deeply but I can't do anything about it. When I am over medicated no one wants to be around me.

Now comes the balance. Now comes the challenge. Now comes the decision. Do I risk making myself feel comfortable but everyone else uncomfortable, or do I risk making myself feel uncomfortable and everyone else comfortable? My outlook on life has always been centered on "me and my needs," so that is the direction I head. I prefer to make myself feel comfortable.

You ask, "What do you do to get over the hump?" There are two divisions in my 24-hour day: sleep time and awake time.

Sleep time is much easier to control. When a Parkinson's patient is sleeping, his symptoms do not appear (this is truly through the grace of God). My only need for medicine is enough to get me up and to the bathroom. Therefore, the amount of dopamine that I pump into my body is much less, but I still need some. So during the night when I wake up (after 3 to 4 hours) I take a pill.

However, my biggest concern is when I near the morning hours. I have to be able to get up and move freely. So, about 30 to 45 minutes before I have to get out of bed I take 2 pills simply to assure that I won't just lay there frozen in my bed like a day-old cadaver. Then throughout the day it's a continuous hit and miss proposition.

Every day that I get up I don't know how my body is going to be hindered by my disease. Each morning I start the same way. When I get up the first thing I do is take a triple play. That's my little code word for the three different medications I take. Individually they are Comtan (nicknamed "the football" or "brownie"), Requip (the "Chrysler" or "pinkie") and Sinemet the ("yellow pill").

When I ask Kathy or my mom for any of these they know exactly what to get me. Fifteen to twenty minutes after I have taken my first triple play, if I don't see a significant improvement in my symptoms, then I start gobbling down pills until I do. I don't really gobble them down haphazardly, but I do start taking Sinemet (dopamine) one at a time or alternate with another drug until I am free of my bonds. The truth be known, I would rather be over-medicated than under-medicated.

And so that is the battle I will face for the rest of my life.

6

THE BALLWASHER INTRO

THE BALLWASHER INTRO

THE GRIPS

As I said, one of the problems that I have had from early on with Par-kinson's has been the strength of my grip. It primarily affects my left hand. In fact, at one point it was so bad I gave up the game of golf. It was no longer fun for me. I usually shoot in the mid-90's (a bogey golfer), but I was shooting 120-plus. The reason was that I could not hold on to the clubs anymore: they kept turning in my hand. I could hit every shot the pros hit: a hook, a slice, a fade, and a draw—the only difference is I had no idea when I was going to hit them.

Regretfully, I told my buddy Bill that I wasn't going play anymore and the reason why. He said that he understood, but wished there was some other answer. The next day while eating dinner, Bill called and said he had a solution. He suggested that I replace my current grips with training grips (pre-formed grips to help inexperienced golfers hold the club properly). I said that sounds fine, but those grips are illegal. He said, "Who cares, I want you to play golf with me. Besides, you're the only one I can consistently beat."

So the next morning I went down to the golf shop and replaced all my grips. I was excited and anxious. I wanted to swing my clubs. I called Bill at his office and asked him if he wanted to go to the driving range with me so I could try out my "new" clubs. He of course said yes. So when I got home I changed my clothes, picked up Bill, and off we went.

The new grips did not fit my hands the way my old grips did and I was concerned how I would hit the ball. "That's stupid" I thought to myself, "it can't be any worse than you are hitting them now." The first 10-15 balls went all over the place. I couldn't hit a thing. Bill said, maybe I was trying too hard: "Slow down and just make a nice smooth swing." I took his advice.

My next shot was a pretty nice drive. I slowed down my tempo again and hit another nice shot. Could these grips be my salvation? I sure hoped so. I finished hitting my bucket of balls, and for the most part I hit them fairly well. The true test would be when I actually played a round of golf. When we got home I called my favorite golf course, North Kent, and made a tee time for 8:00 A.M. Bill said he would take the following day off so he could play with me (don't get too misty eyed with his generous offer-he's self-employed). The next day could not come fast enough.

"This is it" I thought … I stood on the #1 tee with my driver in hand. Boy was I nervous. Bill said, "Remember your tempo."

I took a deep breath, let it out, started my back swing, and took a nice swipe at the ball. It rolled ten feet in front of me. Bill commented, "Nice shot, Money" (Bill's nickname for me, though I can't remember where it came from). I picked up my ball, re-teed it, and took another nice swing. I hit a beautiful drive.

As we played on, my subsequent shots were sporadic but overall, I was pleased. After finishing the round I wish I could tell you my game was fantastic, but it wasn't. I shot a 52, however a 52 was much better than the 60's I had been shooting. I had hope.

Over the next couple of weeks I worked diligently on my swing and was able to bring it back to the way it was. I was very thankful to Bill. I could still play the sport that I loved. I have used these grips ever since. I explain to new playing partners why I have the grips and no one has said a thing about it; they are just glad that I am playing again.

THE BALLWASHER

As my Parkinson's has progressed my inability to grip and hold on to things has increased substantially. I have spilled so many beverages and plates of food on our family room carpet that it looks similar to a Picasso painting. It's even hard to tell what the original color was.

One of the last vacations that Kathy and I took was to Lexington, KY. Our intent was to play some golf, go to Keeneland, see some sights, and just relax. The first three days we did exactly that. Kathy used to be a very good golfer but recently has given up on the game. Now she enjoys just riding along with me to keep me company and harass me when I hit a bad shot (which is far more often than I would like).

I had played golf on a different course everyday while on vacation. I enjoy playing on different golf courses because each offers me a new challenge and every course has its individual beauty. I don't think I would like belonging to a country club because playing the same course every day would drive me nuts (plus I could never afford it).

On the fourth day of our vacation I asked Kathy if I could play golf later that afternoon. She said sure, and that she would like to join me, so we called down to the front desk and asked the concierge for some recommendations for another course in the area. He recommended a newer 18-hole course that had just opened last season and was supposed to be very nice. He offered to make us a tee time, but I said it wasn't necessary as it was the middle of the week and I was sure the course wasn't crowded. So, we headed out.

Upon arriving at the course I was amazed to see the parking lot was full. I couldn't believe it. "I hope we can get out," I told Kathy and proceeded to go into the pro shop. I went up to the counter and asked the gentleman if I could get out. He said I couldn't play 18 holes, as he had an outing going on, but if I was interested in just playing nine holes I could play the front nine. I said that would be fine.

As a courtesy, and to save myself an embarrassing situation (having someone think that I was sneaking Kathy on to the course without paying), I always advised the starter that my wife would be joining me for just the ride. He said that would be no problem at all, but they charged $8. I said, "You have to be kidding," and he replied, "No, that's our policy." So I paid the $8 and headed out the door. I climbed in the golf cart and drove over to the car and started to load up the clubs.

I told Kathy that I couldn't believe it, but they charged $8 for her to ride along. She replied, "Does he think we are some kind of idiots? I'm not paying $8." (I thought to myself, I must be a real idiot because I just did.), I'm going to go shopping instead. Make sure you get our money back, (I always get instructions.) I put up a brief struggle, but learned long ago not to argue with Kathy.

So, I told her to be back in about 2 ½ hours, got in the golf cart, and drove back to the clubhouse. When I walked into the pro shop I could see that the manager was quite busy. I asked him if I could get my $8 back because my wife wasn't coming along after all. He said that would not be a problem, but asked if I could come back after my round was over and get it then, as he was extremely busy with the outing. When I said that was fine, he let out a little sigh of relief, and I headed to the first tee.

The layout of the first hole was spectacular. If the rest of this course was anything like this first hole, this was going to be a gorgeous course to play. It appeared as if it was carved right out of the forest. If you hooked or sliced you were in big trouble. The fairways were fairly wide and gave some relief for the errant shot but not enough. I lit a cigar, put on my golf glove, and walked up to the tee box. I hammered a 260-yard drive right down the center of the fairway. I was turned on; this was going to be a great day. I put my second shot eight feet from the cup and rolled in the putt for a birdie. What a way to start.

As I played on, every hole was the same. It was majestic, colorful, and serene. On the fourth hole, where the green was not too far from a lake, a six-point buck walked right across the green in front of me. I stood there mesmerized as I watched this magnificent creature walk majestically across the green. I thought to myself, "This is one of the few golf courses I would like to play all the time."

When I hit my second shot on #5 it landed in the trap on the right side of the green. As I drove along the edge of the fairway I saw the path to the #6 tee. I thought I saw the tee box to the right and made a mental note of it. I chipped onto the green, putted out, and hopped in the cart and zipped over to the next tee box.

As I raced through the cutaway to the #6 tee, I remembered seeing the tee box to the right. I was playing very well, it was a beautiful day, and I was excited. I was driving much faster than I should have. As I turned to the right to go to the tee box, I quickly discovered that these were the forward tees. Without slowing down, I made a crucial error, a blunder, a faux pas. I swung hard to the left, and as I made the turn, I lost my grip on the wheel. It slipped completely out of my hands (I had a brief flashback of my Mother saying "John … Please don't ride no-handed"), and I lost TOTAL control of the golf cart.

Right in front of me was a brand new ball washing machine. I let out a howl like the cry of a Banshee and then, "NOOOOOO!" as I smashed into the ball washer head on and chopped it off at ground level. Pieces were flying all over the place.

If that wasn't bad enough, by the time I had found the brake pedal I was right on top of a brand new oak (hard as cement) and Plexiglas diagram of the hole. I hit the frame hard—very hard. The Plexiglas shattered and flew everywhere. But that wasn't the only thing that flew. I shot out of the front of the cart like the human cannonball at the circus. "I can fly!" ... Well maybe, but it was no three-point landing (If you've ever seen film of a dodo bird landing ... BINGO). I took temporary notice that there were no seat belts in the cart. But then again, why in God's name should there be?

Upon impact the cart stalled and came to a stop. I sat there, ashamed, scared, and angry for all the damage I had done. At least the beautiful oak frame was still standing.

Then I heard this ungodly squeaking sound followed by a kind of crunching sound. My eyes were drawn to the frame. I thought I saw a little movement. Oh my God, I did see movement. The beautiful oak frame came crashing to the ground. What was I going to do now? I was lying in a heap but unhurt. I looked at the front of my golf cart. It was shattered, with a hole the size of a softball missing in front, but thankfully it still ran. I thought for several minutes of what to do. I decided that since there was nothing anyone could do now, I would finish my round and would tell the manager after my round was over. I really am a possessed golfer.

The next three holes were disastrous to say the least, I scattered balls everywhere. When I walked off the 9th green, I was exhausted, anxious, and a little scared. How was I going to tell the manager what happened, but most importantly, how was he going to react? When I walked up to the clubhouse I saw Kathy sitting in the parking lot. I waved to her and she waved back. I held up my finger—noooo ... my index finger, indicating I needed a minute.

As I entered the pro shop I could see that the outing was over, and most everyone had left. That was a big relief to me. The last thing I wanted to do was to tell the manager that I pulverized everything that was standing on the 6th tee in front of a hundred drunks.

After telling my story to the owner about having Parkinson's, losing my grip, and wiping out his ball washer and hole diagram sign, I braced for the blow—which never came. He couldn't have been nicer (ahhhh that Southern hospitality). He told me to wait a minute while he called his insurance agent. After a brief conversation of, "Uhuh, yea, uhuh, ok, and ok," he came back to me and said that the insurance would cover everything but the deductible and he would be happy to split it with me. That was it. As I walked back to the car, my eyes were directed towards Kathy. I could tell right away that she was upset for being kept waiting so long. Now terror really struck: I had to recount the entire story to her.

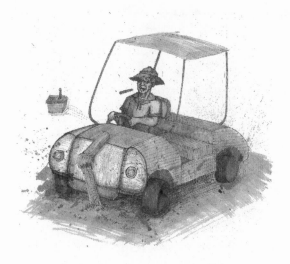

7

THE DRIVE

THE DRIVE

DROWSINESS

All the warnings of drowsiness that one finds on allergy, cold, and other medicines has never concerned me. Drowsiness, in the past has never affected me. That is why, when I noted the same warning on my Parkinson's medication Amantadine, I paid no attention to it. I soon discovered that it did affect me and that I can fall asleep at the drop of a hat—sitting, standing, or eating—anytime, anywhere, except at bedtime when I want to go to sleep.

One of the gifts of life that has been bestowed upon me (and believe me there haven't been many) is the ability to laugh at myself and find humor in almost anything.

At this particular time I was employed by a hotel management company. My job function was two-fold. I was the General Manager of a hotel in Grand Rapids, MI, and also acted as an area manager by assisting and directing Bob Kolomak, the General Manager of our Saginaw property.

On a sunny day in July I had scheduled a visit to Saginaw. It was generally a 2 ½ to 3 hour drive. I had not slept well that night (which was becoming more of a recurring irritant). I ate breakfast, swallowed a couple of Amatadines, and headed out the door. It was 7:00 A.M.

About an hour and a half into the drive I started feeling sleepy. I should have pulled over and stopped at a rest area or a restaurant parking lot and taken a short nap (which I always do now). But I didn't. As I said, becoming drowsy behind the wheel had never been a problem for me before, and so far I was able to shake it off. Becoming ever more sleepy, I rolled down the window, turned up the radio, and began singing loudly. A bird wasn't seen for miles and you could hear the painful howl of neighborhood dogs but I carried on. My singing voice gets the same reaction in people as fingernails on a chalkboard. I crooned for a while longer and then couldn't stand myself any more. I rolled up the windows, turned down the radio, and told myself I would be all right. WRONG!

One of the very few faults I have is that I am a fast and impatient driver. As I was heading east on I-69 at 75 mph, I came upon an *idiot* who was driving a red Lincoln 65 mph in the left hand passing lane. This knucklehead was driving next to another car (who was in the right hand lane) but would not pass him. He just stayed there, blocking both lanes. I came upon him very rapidly, and rode his rear-end for several miles, but he wouldn't move over. It finally became apparent to me that this guy was a real jerk and must have gotten some kind of perverse pleasure out of doing this. He was not going to move over easily. "Well, Mr. Red Lincoln I'm not done yet," I thought.

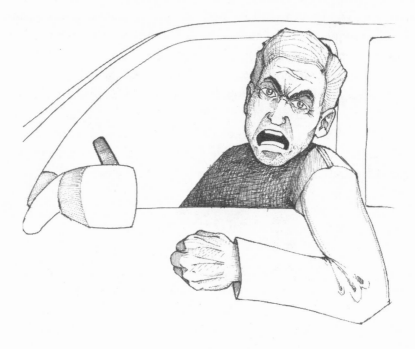

I accelerated, rode his rear-end again, and laid on the horn. When I saw him look in his rear view mirror I raised my hand and I showed him that he was number one. He must have been a very conceited person because he showed me that he agreed. I was ready to pop my cork. It was obvious I was getting nowhere!

In order to avoid giving myself a stroke or a heart attack, I backed off a little but still stayed close. This SOB was not going to move over. I continued like this for some time, but I started feeling drowsy again. Then the nods set in. Let me tell you, this is your last warning sign, and you had better take notice. Then it happened: I became very, very drowsy, and I told myself I would close my eyes for just a second. That little voice spoke to me … "YOU SHOULDN'T DO THAT JOHN."

BUMP, BUMP, BANG, BUMP, THUMP. WHAT THE HELL??????? AAAAARRRRGGGGGHHH!

When I opened my eyes I found myself down in the grassy median doing 65 miles per hour … ASLEEP!

Fill your pants, call in your tokens, it's time to meet your maker … ATTENTION!

What happened next took only seconds but seemed like minutes. I glanced up at the highway and couldn't believe what I was seeing. If I wasn't petrified and scared to death, I would have broken into hysterical laughter. Mr. Red Lincoln was hanging out the window with his eyes bulging out of his head. It looked like somebody had stuck two ping-pong balls with little black dots on his forehead.

He slowed up, and in that instinctive moment I stepped on the accelerator, turned right, and up the embankment I went, passing him in a cloud of dust and hearty HI-O silver. In my rearview mirror I watched him move over to the right lane and I never saw that jerk again.

I let out a chuckle every time I picture this guy telling his friends, "And this lunatic must have gotten fed up, and I swear to God, he passed me in the median …"

8

BALANCE

BALANCE

During the first few years of my battle with Parkinson's, balance was never anything that I was concerned with. Since then, however, it has become a major issue. I fall or stumble all the time. Loss of balance is a symptom of Parkinson's and one that most patients have to deal with.

My Parkinson's doctor, Dr. Neuman, is very well respected and tops in his field. His concern and concentration while examining his patients is appreciated by all of us (except when I crack a joke and get no response). One such occurrence happened while we were discussing balance and it was the first time the subject had been brought up. Dr. Neuman asked me, "John, are you starting to fall alot?" Being the quick wit that I am, I responded "No more than usual." ... ZOOOM ... He didn't even crack a smile. That really hurt.

The general areas where I have trouble with my balance are when I am standing for an extended period of time. My inclination is to start backing up and I cannot stop myself until I run in to something and fall to the floor. The other area is when I have a sudden shift of my weight from one side to the other. Doing this will result in disaster. I have to be totally aware of where I am and what I am doing at all times in order to prevent myself from being seriously hurt. Following are three instances concerning balance.

THE JUNKYARD

One evening I decided to organize the "junkyard." Most people call it a basement. Every year our subdivision has a huge garage sale and this year I was bound and determined that we were going to get rid of some of the stuff down there. We had lived in our house nine years and there were boxes in the junkyard that had never been opened. There was junk everywhere. I hadn't seen my basement floor in years.

It was about 3:00 A.M. and I couldn't sleep. I had been working in the junkyard for two or three hours and I was getting a little winded and fatigued. I wanted to sit down, but there was stuff strewn everywhere and nowhere to sit, so I decided I would just stand there for a few moments and catch my breath. I couldn't have been there for more than two minutes and suddenly I started to feel myself lean backwards. OH OH, I immediately knew this wasn't good. I took a step backwards, and then another, and another ... there was no stopping me now. I kept backing up until I hit my golf bag that was lying on the floor.

I flew through the air with the greatest of ease and fell into a charcoal grill and smashed against the wall and dropped to the ground in a heap. I laid there for several minutes to catch my breath and tried to determine if I had broken anything. I had hit the wall very hard but I was fairly sure that I was still in one piece. I thought to myself, "You are one lucky guy, you could have hurt yourself very seriously." I dusted myself off and decided to call it a night and went to bed.

THE SEWER DISPLAY

When Kathy and I moved to the Grand Rapids, MI area we were look-ing for a new home in a nice area. We found such a home in Rockford, MI. The community has a quaint ambiance and a very cute down-town. The downtown consists of restaurants, gift shops, antique shops, and one-of-a-kind shops. In addition to this (as if anything could be any better), there is a river that runs right through the center of town that harbors trout and salmon. (Norman Rockwell, eat your heart out.) We found a very nice home for sale about one mile from downtown with a double lot.

I've always wanted a house on a large lot so I couldn't say yes to the deal fast enough. The one thing I wasn't nuts about was that in the backyard was a storm sewer. It was a city ordinance that it should be there and be kept open. In my opinion it was an eyesore. I didn't like it at all.

I was sitting on my deck one August afternoon staring at my beauti-ful storm sewer. A flash of brilliance suddenly came over me. If it couldn't be removed, perhaps it could it be hidden! In the corner of our lot was a steep hill that surrounded the sewer on three sides. If the city would allow me to dig out a large planting bed at the bottom, dig up the hill about four feet, and terrace it all the way around the hill, it could be something quite awe-inspiring.

I put together a diagram of what I intended to do, which included a computerized shrub, flower, and bush layout. I took it down to city hall. Hallelujah! Virginia, there is a Santa Claus … it was approved. I started to convert it the very next day.

To make a long story short, the "sewer display" (this is how Kathy and I refer to it today) was transformed into a thing of beauty. It is now the focal point of our backyard. You would never know that it disguised that ugly sewer.

When working in the sewer display I need to be very careful. There are three levels, each separated from the others by a row of large boulders. This is not only decorative but it prevents erosion as well. It also makes an excellent place for me to spill my brains out all over the rocks if I'm not careful. Directly surrounding the sewer are four variegated dogwood bushes. These bushes grow thick, grow fast, and grow tall. In the spring it is necessary for me to cut them back to the height of about two feet.

One of the symptoms of Parkinson's that I have struggled with for some time now has been my balance, because it comes and goes. I don't know what triggers it because it doesn't seem to be a problem for me all the time. But when I have trouble with it, I am continually falling.

For my safety I almost always sit down when I'm in the sewer display. I either sit on the boulders, on my stool, or on the ground. One afternoon I decided to do some weeding on the terraces. I took my stool, and (as always) started on the top level and worked my way down.

I was there about 15 minutes when an annoying little honeybee decided he wanted my spot. After several unsuccessful attempts at trying to shoo him away, my patience wore thin. When he came at me again, I grabbed my trowel, and decided I was going to bean the little bugger.

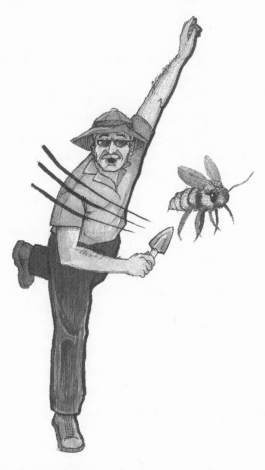

When
he got close enough I reeled back, and with all my force took a mighty
swipe at the little bee. (JOHN, YOU SHOULDN'T HAVE SWUNG
SO HARD that little voice shouted.) Not only did I miss the little
honeybee by a mile, but also the force of that swing caused me to lose
my balance and dive head first into the sewer display.

It's funny how quick the mind can react. I braced myself for the
intense pain I was about to feel. However, the pain I felt was not the
bone-bruising pain I expected; instead it was a sharp (and I mean

sharp), stinging pain all over my body. I had just performed a 1-½ gainer in the layout position into the dogwood bushes. To my utter amazement I never hit the ground. I landed upside-down, with my right arm pinned behind my back, head straight down, and my feet dangling out of the variegated dogwood bushes.

Two things should be noted *now* that were totally unimportant *before* I entered the sewer display but were vitally important now: 1) I needed my medication soon—I began to feel tremors in my hands and my legs were beginning to stiffen up; and 2) I never do well upside-down.

As I remained suspended there my thoughts went to how lucky I was that a branch didn't poke my eye out, or even worse—that I didn't break my neck. After dwelling on this for about thirty seconds, panic began to creep in. My thoughts went instantly to "WHAT IN THE HELL AM I GOING TO DO NOW?"

I tried to move my right arm. Impossible. I could not budge it. I tried to move my left arm. I could move it quite far, but when I did it caused one of the branches to dig deep into my side. "WHAT IN THE HELL AM I GOING TO DO NOW?" As I thought of what I must look like to those passing by on the sidewalk, I started to laugh. The more I laughed the louder I got. The louder I got the more I laughed. Bordering on hysteria I imagined how utterly ridiculous I must look and sound upside down in those bushes. Thank God none of the neighbors came walking by at that particular moment, as they surely would have hauled me off to the funny farm without a second thought.

"John," I said to myself, "in a very short time this isn't going to be funny ... Get a hold of yourself." I didn't have a lot of options and it didn't require a brain surgeon to determine what I had to do next. I had to get someone over here fast and help me get out.

There was only one way to do that ... scream for help. I took a deep breath and started to scream at the top of lungs, "HEEEELP ... HEEEEELP ... HEEEEEEELP!" I yelled and I yelled until I was blue in the face, which was pretty hard to do seeing my face was beet red from being upside down for so long. No one came.

After several minutes of this I gave up. I wasn't getting anywhere. My throat was sore and I was exhausted. The situation was not looking good. I still hung there upside-down. Now I started to feel real panicky. The shakes were getting worse. I was starting to get very stiff, and I was beginning to think my head was going to pop from the pressure of the blood that had rushed to it. Remember that game we had as kids, Mr. Potato Head? Now they could have a new game and name it after me: Mr. Tomato Head.

Well as I hung there upside down in a tangle of branches with a red head, a raspy voice, and shaking like hell, I could only think of one thing: "Please God don't let Kathy come home and find me like this. She will never leave me home alone again." That's when reality finally set in. In a moment of utter brilliance, I came to the conclusion that the only way I was going to get out of this mess was to do it myself.

I thought carefully about what I had to do. First, with my left arm I was going to reach as far down as I could and grab the biggest branch and pull with all my might. Second, although I couldn't do much with my right arm, I was going to push as hard as I could. Lastly, I was going to turn, twist, rock, or do the Mamba—whatever it took to get me to the ground.

"Are we ready gang? Then let's go." And with that, I pushed, pulled, turned, twisted, rocked and danced the Mamba. The pain was terrible, but I didn't stop until I felt myself go plunk on the ground. I hurt badly, I was a bloody mess, and I was totally exhausted, but it felt great! I was on the ground.

As I lay there I looked up the hill and saw the little honeybee land gently on one of my yellow double marigolds. The little bastard!

GREEN KNEES AND TP

Another incident regarding balance happened to me about four years ago. I was invited to attend a very exclusive golf outing. The participants, for the most part, were presidents and CEO's of local corporations. There were several pro golfers who would also be in attendance. I was very excited to be part of this event, and on top of that, it didn't cost me a dime.

I was there because my best friend Pat Tinetti was organizing the event. Once again that old adage "it's not what you know ... it's whom you know" was proven correct. If the truth were known, I actually believe he had some cancellations and had no one else to call. I didn't care ... I was there.

I couldn't wait for our foursome to be assigned. I asked Pat if I could be paired up with a pro. He called a week before the outing and told me it wasn't going to happen. The pros were playing with the big contributors. Well, that certainly left me out. I was a little disappointed but that didn't dampen my enthusiasm. This was a first class golf outing. The golf course was outstanding. The meal being served consisted of hors d'oeuvres, a salad bar, and sirloin strips with all the sides. In addition to that there was an open bar. There would also be door prizes and awards.

I wanted my equipment to look good so I washed and polished my clubs. It had been a long time since I had done that, they were filthy. I scrubbed and cleaned my golf bag, too. I bought two dozen new golf balls, a couple bags of tees, new head covers, and two new golf gloves.

That was it from an equipment standpoint. Everything was either clean or new and everything was looking good. However, the most difficult task still lay ahead of me—selecting what I was going to wear. This was a big event. Most of the golfers made ten times the salary I made so $95.00 golf shirts were not going to be uncommon; although you wouldn't find one in my closet.

I wanted to look good. I have absolutely no taste and cannot coordinate two colors unless one of the colors is white. Therefore, it was necessary for me to consult my fashion designer, Kathy.

Over dinner, I reminded Kathy that I was playing in a golf outing Thursday and asked for her assistance in choosing my outfit. She reluctantly said she would, but didn't understand why, as I never listen to what she has to say. I opted not to respond and let it pass.

After dinner I began my fashion show. All I needed was a runway and some floor lights and one would have thought they were at a premier fashion show on Fifth Avenue. For over an hour and a half I came in and out of the bedroom, each time wearing a different look. I paraded in front of Kathy, took swings with an invisible golf club, stood still, and even twirled.

Finally, Kathy said "Stop … I can't do this anymore. I thought I would just have to go into your closet and pick out something for you to wear. This is nuts! I've already told you that three or four of the outfits you've "modeled" looked very nice, but you keep coming out with more and more. I'm going to bed."

"Please don't," I begged. "I only have three left to try on."

Kathy hemmed and hawed for a minute and then finally said "Ok, but make it quick."

After another twenty-five minutes the show was over. I had to admit I was pretty tired too.

"Kathy, which one did you like best?" She told me that any of the four she had previously mentioned looked very nice on me.

"John, I'm going to sleep in the spare bedroom tonight so you can put away every piece of clothing that you've taken out. Good night."

Kathy would have strangled me if she knew what I was contemplating. How was I going to pull this off? I wanted her to pick out the clothes that absolutely looked the best on me. I didn't want something that just looked good; I wanted something that looked fantastic and very expensive too. I wanted to tell her that tomorrow night I was going to try on those four outfits again, and I wanted her to pick out the very best one. I hated to be a pain in the rear but this golf outing was big, really big, and I wanted to look sharp.

I knew *I* couldn't pick out the best looking outfit, in fact the one I liked best (I will admit was a little wild) was a pair of lime green slacks, a lime green and pink striped shirt, a white hat and white golf shoes. When I came walking out of the bedroom in that attire and told Kathy that I really liked it … she said, "You've got to be kidding. If you so much as even think about wearing those ridiculous looking clothes to the outing I'll never speak to you again. Furthermore, you look like a giant kiwi."

The following night we had a nice dinner. After we finished eating, I cleaned up, and helped wash the dishes. I was a little nervous about asking Kathy to partake in another fashion show, but I have no taste, and therefore I had no choice.

I hit her with the question … to my surprise and delight she said she would be happy to do it … she understood I just wanted to look my best in front of all those big shots. So, once again, I tried on the four outfits she liked. When I was done Kathy selected … khaki slacks, a brown and beige striped golf shirt, a brown sleeveless sweater, brown and tan golf shoes and my beige Pebble Beach hat ... done!

Tomorrow was the big day and I was geeked. I laid out my clothes and put my clubs and shoes by the front door. I was all set. I had never played this course before (its private) but I knew where it was. It should take about twenty to thirty minutes to get there. I planned on leaving about 9:00 A.M., which would give me plenty of spare time ... (Or so I thought).

As I got into bed, I said a little prayer to the golf gods to please let me hit them long and straight tomorrow, kissed Kathy good night, rolled over, and fell asleep.

I reached over the bed and shut off the alarm (God that's an awful sound). I felt very rested. I laid there for a few moments and then got out of bed. It was 7:15 AM. Kathy was already up and was downstairs cooking breakfast. The smell of bacon and coffee drifted upstairs.

I got out of the shower, dried off, slapped some shaving cream on my face, and grabbed my razor. On the fourth stoke I felt a stinging sensation on my chin. I gazed into the mirror. Then I saw it. It started as a little red speck, but started growing larger. I blotted it with some tissue again and again but it wouldn't stop bleeding. I am not a hemophiliac but I don't stop bleeding very easily.

I tore off a small piece of tissue and stuck it on my gash. I finished shaving, got dressed in my golf clothes, and went downstairs into the kitchen. When Kathy turned around she blurted out "What happened to you?" I told her that I had nicked myself shaving. "It looks like you did more than just nick your chin," she responded. "It's bleeding pretty badly."

"Does it look terrible?" I asked. "Kind of," she replied. "But give it a little time, it will stop. Why don't you sit down and eat your breakfast."

I am normally not much of a breakfast eater, but this morning I was starving. We chatted for a few minutes and then Kathy said she had to get going, as she didn't want to be late for work. I said, "Ok, I just want you to know, I'm thinking of not going to the outing with this bloody chin."

Kathy snapped at me. "Don't be foolish, you've been looking forward to this event ever since you were invited. Your wound will dry up … you go and have a great time. I love you, Goodbye." With that she was out the door and gone. It was 8:05 A.M.

I went into the bathroom and pulled off the piece of red tissue paper dangling from my chin. Damn … it was still bleeding. I opened up the medicine cabinet and looked for a small bandage. There weren't any, only the large finger size. Well, I sure wasn't going to use one of those; it would cover my whole chin. I would just leave a little earlier, stop at the drug store, and buy some smaller ones. I tore off a larger piece of TP and stuck it on my chin.

The breakfast Kathy made for me was very good but I was still hungry. It was 8:20 A.M. I didn't have a lot of time to waste. I opened the refrigerator and saw an opened package of bacon. Did I have time to cook some more? Sure, I thought to myself, if you hurry. So I grabbed a frying pan, turned the burner on high and plopped four or five strips of bacon in the pan. They started to sizzle and pop almost immediately. I looked for my splatter screen (It's a utensil that prevents grease from splattering all over the place. While in college I was watching an infomercial and decided I just had to have one) but I couldn't find it now. So, there I stood with grease splattering and turned the bacon.

After about ten minutes, the bacon was crispy and done. I gobbled it down. It was 8:30 A.M. I was all set and ready to go. I took my clubs and shoes out to the car and put them in the trunk. I got in the car and put the key in the ignition. I turned the key but it didn't start ... in fact it didn't turn over.

Oh no ... don't tell me ... please this can't be happening.

That little man in my head spoke up, "You idiot ... you left your headlights on last night didn't you? Your battery is dead."

"Who are you Mr. Goodwrench?" I mumbled, but I knew he was right. When I got home yesterday I must have forgotten to turn the lights off.

What was I going to do now?

I needed a jump-start but whom could I call? All of my neighbors worked, so I was sure I wouldn't find anyone at home, but I thought I better try anyway ... so I raced up-stairs, grabbed our telephone book, and began to call everyone on the block. As I suspected, no one was home. It was now 8:50 A.M.

What was I going to do now?

That little voice interrupted, "I don't know numbskull, but I'll tell you one thing, if you don't leave soon you are going to be late for the outing and your buddy is counting on you being there."

I called the local service station for some roadside assistance and explained my predicament to the gentleman on the phone. He assured me that they would send someone over as soon as possible. I sat in the kitchen and poured myself a cup of cold coffee, watched the clock, and waited. It was 9:05 A.M. I had less than an hour.

At 9:30 A.M. I was a nervous wreck. I was becoming uneasy and I was getting angry. No one had come yet. As I picked up the phone to dial the service station I saw the wrecker coming down the street. I hung up the phone, grabbed my wallet, locked the door and raced outside to meet him.

As I ran across the front lawn I suddenly felt something odd with my legs. They felt heavy. They were not doing what I expected them to do. I thought I was running sideways. My balance left me. I was struggling to stay on my feet. But alas, that was not going to happen. On a full run, I went flying through the air (not at all like Superman), landed in a praying position, and dug both knees into the sod.

The mechanic came running over to see if I was all right. I told him I was OK, but to please go back and finish jumping my car. When I got to my feet I looked down at my knees. I was staring at the biggest grass stains I had ever seen. My slacks were a mess. I didn't have time to worry about that now ... get the car started first and then go back to the house and change. *Any* clothes as long as they were clean would be fine now (except the lime green outfit). How quickly we change our priorities.

The mechanic finished connecting the cables and told me to try and start the car. I got in but I couldn't find my keys, I must have left them in the house ... that's OK I told myself as I always carry an extra car key in my wallet. I got it out and put it in the ignition. Vrrrooooom.... it started right up. I reiterated that I was in hurry and gave him my credit card. He quickly filled out the bill, we exchanged thank you's and he drove away. It was 9:45 AM. I was definitely going to be late.

I left the car running, (I had to change very fast), ran up to the front door, and turned the handle and pushed—OH *MY GOD, IT'S LOCKED!* I ran to the back of the house and tried that door ... LOCKED. I stood there dumbfounded. I had absolutely no idea of what to do next. I stumbled and almost fell again.

POOF the little man spoke again, "Johnny boy, you have NO time to waste, you are already going to be late. You may think you have several options but you don't. You only have two ... GO or DON'T GO. If you choose the latter you will let down your best friend, screw up a foursome, and miss out on the fun. If you go ... granted you look a mess, but you've learned to laugh at yourself, people will understand, and in spite of everything you will still have a good time."

I opened the door, got in the car, and drove away. It was 9:55 A.M.

As I was driving, I thought about what could take place when I arrived at the golf course. To my delight, I could only come up with two scenarios and both were good news. 1) If they teed off late because people were eating or still visiting I could slip into the pro shop and quickly buy a pair of slacks and meet my partners on our first hole or 2) If they had already teed off, I could still buy a pair of slacks, and join my team on the second hole. In either case, only a handful of people might see me ... I could deal with that. I started feeling much better.

I made it to the golf course in twenty-two minutes. That little man blurted out "Way to go Dale Earnhardt." I parked the car, grabbed my clubs, threw them over my shoulder, and ran across the parking lot. As I rounded the corner of the huge clubhouse (panting heavily with my golf clubs clinking and clanking) ... I immediately discovered there was a third scenario ... That everyone would be lined up be sitting in their carts, smack dab in front of me, listening to a welcoming speech from Pat.

I froze dead in my tracks. There I stood in front of everyone with khaki pants and green knees. All eyes were focused on me. Pat turned his attention to me and announced, "This is my best friend John … glad to see you could make it … nice pants."

There was an uproar of laughter and I joined in. He turned away from the microphone and said, "Where have you been? I'm almost finished. Stay right there and I'll get you hooked up with your foursome. When he finished his speech, everyone started their carts and headed for their designated tee-off hole. Unfortunately everyone had to pass by me. As they did most were still chuckling and several were pointing. Pat's line was funny, but it wasn't that funny.

Pat came over as my team members pulled up in their carts. He introduced my playing partners to me and then pulled me aside "What happened to you … you look a mess?"

"Pat, it's a long story" I replied.

"Did you cut yourself shaving?" he asked.

"Yes I did. Does it look bad?"

"Well it would look a hell of lot better if you didn't have that red hunk of tissue hanging off your chin."

Whaaat? I reached up, felt the piece of TP, and removed it. In my frenzied state, I had forgotten about the TP on my chin and stopping at the drug store for a bandage.

"Couldn't you find a clean sweater, either?" he asked.

I looked down and couldn't believe my eyes. All over the front of my sweater were stains ... ***THE BACON*** ... the grease had splattered all over the front of my sweater.

I thought for a moment of when I had first arrived, and shuddered ... Standing there in front of everybody with two gigantic grass stained knees, a wad of red TP hanging from my chin, and wearing a grease-soaked sweater. That little man chortled, "I bet everyone thought your outfit looked fantastic and expensive too!"

"Boy, he could be a pain in the butt" I thought.

Pat you won't believe what's happened to me today ... I don't believe it myself. I don't have time to tell you now, so I'll catch you later this afternoon. I got in the cart with my playing partner and we drove off.

I looked like crap, but that didn't matter anymore. The embarrassment was over (or so I thought). The most important thing now was to just have a good time.

My team members were very nice men. We had an afternoon of laughs, many at my expense as I retold the happenings of my day. We simply had a great time. My partners were bogey golfers just like me. This meant we could either end up winning the whole thing or coming in last place. You just never knew.

We started off pretty well. Our first hole was the number three-handicap hole (third hardest on the course). I rolled in a nice seven-foot putt for a par. On the second hole we all hit our drives. I hit a boomer right down the center of the fairway. They all let oooos and aaahhs and gave me a little ovation. I was feeling better ... everything was going to be all right.

We drove to my ball. As I went to get out of the cart my legs felt funny, like they did earlier in the day. My right leg dragged and I caught one of my cleats on the edge of the cart. I shot out of the cart like a rocket, arms flailing wildly with my head down. I raced across the fairway at lighting speed. Have you ever seen a trumpeter swan try to take off from the water with its wings flapping, head stretched out, and tiptoeing across the water? That's exactly how I looked. The only difference was the swan takes off—I went *SPLAT.*

When I got to my to my feet, I looked at my teammates. They had their backs to me, were bent over and shaking uncontrollably. I was so embarrassed. I felt like a total klutz. Then I pictured myself rocketing out of the golf cart, arms flapping and taking a nosedive into the fairway. I started to laugh hysterically too. We had a great time the rest of the day.

When we finished our round we headed back to the clubhouse for the festivities. The food was excellent and the camaraderie was even better. I didn't win any prizes which I was thankful for—I didn't want to walk up in front of everybody and show-off my "special outfit". All in all, I had a very nice day.

It was finally time to leave. I said my good-byes, grabbed my clubs, and went out to my car. I tossed my clubs in the trunk, got in, and started the car ... *DEAD* ... I just sat there, disgusted. I couldn't believe it. What else could go wrong?

That little man spoke up, "Well mallet-head, in your case, it could be just about anything."

"You're a big help," I thought. I got out of the car and went back to the clubhouse.

I noted that someone had parked on either side of my car that was going to make jumping my car more difficult.

I looked around and found my cart partner. He was getting ready to leave also. I told him I had a dead battery and asked him if he could give me a jump. He said "no problem" and we left. I told him to follow me out to the parking lot and I'd show him where I was parked.

As we approached my car I said, "That's me right there ... and can you believe it, there must be twenty-five to thirty vacant parking spaces in the lot, and some ass has to park right next to me." He turned to me with an odd expression on his face and said, "That ass is me."

OH GOD ... I DID IT AGAIN!

9

THE GOLF CART

THE GOLF CART

CONFUSION

To an individual whose work requires a great deal of multi-tasking and decision-making, confusion can be one of the most devastating symptoms of all. It can drive you right out of your gourd. You can't remember things that you should, you can't remember what you did last, and you can't decide what you need to do next. People wait and wait for a decision.

I would like to tell you about an event that happened to me dealing with confusion. It could have cost me my life at the time but it is pretty funny now.

My mom always taught me to stop, look, and listen as well as look both ways to avoid being run over by a car. But she never told me how to prevent being run over by a golf cart with no driver.

For the past five years my neighbor, Bill, has invited Kathy and me to play in his mom and dad's golf outing. It is comprised of all their friends and neighbors, was only 9 holes, and was conceived just to have fun. And it was!

About four years ago, Kathy and I were playing in the outing. We were at the course early, waiting to see who our team members were going to be. You never knew who your partners were until the day of the outing. The teams were chosen by Bill's dad Al, and were different every year. Although this was just a fun outing, everyone still wanted to win, so it was important that you were on a good team.

When we were given the team rosters, I couldn't have been happier. I knew two of my teammates quite well (Cal, my neighbor, and Bill's mom, Carol), which was great because I am a card-carrying introvert. I am uncomfortable playing with people I don't know. Cal was a six handicap, which was great for our team, and Carol was just a helluva lot of fun.

Another advantage of having Carol in our foursome was that every year Al teed her group off first so that she was the first one finished and could oversee the prize and dinner arrangements. The last plus for our foursome was that, although I didn't know the fourth member of our group (a very attractive young lady), I determined it would be a very enjoyable afternoon watching her putt.

Carol and I decided to share a cart. There wasn't a cloud in the sky, the temperature was 72 degrees, and we had a twelve-pack of brewskies on ice and a thermos of pre-made Bloody Marys. We were set to go. I was sure it was going to be a great day. Victory was within our reach.

Then BANG-BANG-BANG—my great day went to hell. Cal was late ... where was he? Then I saw him in the back of the parking lot (PHEW! He was my ace in the hole, my ringer, one of the few golfers who played very well). I watched him walk across the parking lot and I thought I detected a limp. "Please Lord it can't be," but alas it was; he was limping. When I went out to meet Cal, he told me he hurt his lower back at work and had trouble swinging a club. He could hardly bend over. I expressed my sympathies and then helped him put his golf bag on his cart. Sheeessshh. So much for the "W".

I went looking for Carol because we would be teeing off soon. When I found her she said there was no need to hurry, Al had changed our tee time to last. That way he knew when she arrived at the club-house, everyone was off the course. He also felt more comfortable with us being last, as we would pick up the markers for longest drive, nearest the pin and other contests.

That was just great. What else could go wrong? I no sooner got that thought out of my head when this woman came up and asked, "Are you Carol and John?" Yes, we replied. "Hi, I'm Tracy's mom. She called me from the course and said her son was sick and she had to go home, and wondered if I could play in her place. So here I am."

"Nice to meet you," I answered, and then thought to myself, "Tracy must have a very handsome father."

Well, after an hour and ten minutes of watching everyone else tee off (that's also an hour and ten minutes of drinking Bloody Mary's and Vodka and tonics), I was feeling no pain.

Finally it was our turn to tee off. We all hit our drives. The sad thing was that I had the best drive. It went about 60 yards straight down the fairway and then duck-hooked into the woods. We played on.

For the next six holes we had our moments of glory, but we had many more moments of disaster. We had played seven holes and we were a plus 3. For those of you who don't play golf, that is terrible.

There was only one thing consistent about our round: I continually had problems setting the brake on my golf cart. It was a REAL pain in the butt. I should have returned it to the clubhouse, but that would have been the intelligent thing to do.

On the # 8 hole I hit a nice drive, but thought it might have been a bit long and had gone in a creek that crossed the fairway. We drove along the fairway but were unable to find my ball. It must have gone in the creek, I thought. We told our other partners that we would join them in a minute, as we wanted to look for my ball. I parked the golf cart on top of a small hill about twenty yards from the creek, set the brake, got out, and started looking for my ball.

I looked for about thirty seconds and then I heard it. I know my partners heard it—in fact, I think everyone in the clubhouse heard it: an ear-piercing scream from Carol, "JOHN LOOK OUT!" I whirled around, only to see our golf cart coming straight down the hill heading for the creek. That damn brake. Confusion took over. I stood there flat-footed, unsure of what to do. I couldn't move. I was dumbfounded. Actions were entering my brain from every direction, but I couldn't sort them out. I just stood there unable to move and make a decision. Carol let out another scream, "John, get out of the way!"

The cart was rolling ever closer to the creek. Time was running out. I can't explain what came over me. Yes I can: It was three Bloody Mary's, two vodka and tonics, and two beers. I felt like Superman and I was going to save the day, but I waited too long to react.

I raced over towards the cart. I positioned myself to be in the center of the carts path. In an effort to time my contact with the cart at just the right moment, I started back peddling. I wanted to slow it down and bring it to a stop before it took a nose-dive into the creek. The last thing I heard as I made contact with the cart was Carol yelling, "JOHN DON'T DO IT … LET IT GO!"

Then, contact. I kept back peddling, slowing my pace, but I was running out of ground. I could feel the immense weight and force the cart was producing. But I was Superman—it couldn't hurt me (I think I actually believed it). As I look back, I would have made it if I only had a little more ground to work with, but as it was I ran out of turf.

I made a final thrust to stop it, but no way. The cart just knocked me down and I let out a loud moan as it ran me over. I thank God I didn't hit my head (actually I couldn't have hit my head because my head was dangling over the bank and was half-submerged in the water). If you ever had the desire to know what it feels like to have a golf cart run over your body, let me tell you—as the axles scrape along your shins, the wheels roll over your arms, and you find yourself gnawing on the bumper ... IT DOESN'T FEEL VERY GOOD. I was totally pinned under the cart with the back of my head in the water.

I truly shudder to think what could have happened if I had landed a mere foot farther back or I had waited a few seconds longer. I might very well have drowned. I couldn't see Carol but I sure could hear her. Carol was screaming, "What do I do, what do I do?" In the calmest and loudest voice I could muster, and not wanting it to sound like a panicky scream, I said, "Carol, get in the cart and back it up." There were also a few expletives that I said, but I feel they are not necessary to print here.

As Carol gingerly climbed into the cart, the extra 115 pounds (in case you ever read this, Carol) didn't make any difference. She slowly backed the cart off me. When it was off me, I got to my feet, breathed a sigh of relief, and looked over at Cal. He was on the other side of the fairway bent over laughing in hysterics. There sure didn't seem to be anything wrong with his back now.

10
THE ENEMY

THE ENEMY

For the ten years that I have had Parkinson's, depression from time to time has tried to rear its ugly head, but I have always refused to let it gain a foothold on my psyche. Now, I am not going to sit here and tell you that I have never been down in the dumps, because I have; that I have never felt sorry for myself, because I have; that I never felt like giving up, because I have.

What I am going to tell you is that life is too short. The time we have to share with our family is not enough. The mornings we wake-up and the sun is shining and the birds are singing are not enough. The laughter and the good times that we spend with our friends are not enough. The moments we spend with a pal (in my case my golden retriever "Tyler") are not enough. So I'll be damned if I'm going to let anyone or anything take this precious time from me.

What I have come to know is that in spite of the difficulties that may confront me, the joys in life (family and friends, hobbies and past-times), and the special things that make life so enjoyable are all still available to me. I just have to seek alternate ways of achieving them.

I have known many who when stricken with grief (of one form or another), spend their whole life angry, depressed, or wallowing in self-pity. This hasn't happened to me nor will I let it. It is a waste of time, time that is lost forever and cannot be reclaimed.

Life doles out many surprises. Some good, and some not so good. Dealing with grief is difficult and affects people in different ways. How grieving is handled and for what period of time is an individual thing. There comes a time however when your sadness must be cast aside and you realize that life must go on. The sooner you can accept what life has dealt you, the sooner you will be able to move on. Without acceptance this can never happen.

The only explanation that I can offer to why bad things happen to good people is that they just do … *period*. I realize that this is simplistic, but it is the only honest answer I have. In addition they happen again and again. So you make the decision. You can live the rest of your time on earth saddened, depressed, angry, and miserable or accept the tragedy for what it is and get on living a good and productive life as best you can.

When it comes to the death of a loved one, I can offer this sentiment: death is inevitable, it will happen to all of us. We cannot evade or avoid it. We have absolutely no control over it. So don't fret about when it will happen … it will happen. So get on with living.

My father, who passed away several years ago, will never die, as long I am alive. I talk about him all the time, sharing precious and humorous moments from the past. He always enjoyed playing in a March Madness pool, so every year I fill out a pool in his name. He was never any good at picking his brackets, and I have followed in his footsteps. My Dad will always be alive in my heart.

That's it except for one last thing ...

HERE IS MY GIFT TO YOU

Push the bad things away in your life. Take that first step out the door. Feel the sunshine on your face, the gentle breeze as it touches your hair, smell the flowers in the air, put on a smile and get on living your life. It is yours to cherish, if you want it.

May your life bring you all the happiness you deserve.

Be happy,
John

11

THE CONTEST

THE CONTEST

CONSTIPATION

What a thing to talk about: my inability to poop. Although it doesn't sound serious, it can be. One of the problems I have with constipation is that I can be a little gassy at inopportune times.

Now I'll tell you a story about an incident that happened at my hotel. It took place on a Sunday morning, after I had been constipated for three days due to a new medication.

Although it was Sunday, I came into work for about an hour to check on things and make sure there were no problems. Mike Bunnell, one of my best clerks, was working the front desk. The lobby was full of people milling around and eating breakfast

Before I left for home I went out to the desk to make sure every-thing was all right. Mike was standing at the counter and in front of him were two guest receipts lying on the desk. I asked Mike what they were for. He told me that these guests had called, said they were check-ing out, and wanted their bills ready. I glanced at the receipts, noticed they were both women, and then my mouth opened before my brain went into gear. "Mikie—How about a little wager? I'll take the woman on the right, Mary, you take the one the left, Susan (the names have been changed to protect the innocent). Whoever has the tallest woman loses ... for a buck." Mike said, "You're on."

God how do I get myself into these things?

As I said, the lobby was full of people. Everyone was talking. Every-one was trying to be heard over someone else's voice; you couldn't hear yourself think. Out of the corner of my eye I saw someone coming up to the desk. At first I thought it was a man because the person was so tall … but it wasn't a man it was a woman. As she got closer to the desk she got taller. "Please don't be Mary," I said to myself. When she approached the desk my eyes were wide open and I was starting to feel a little giddy; I had never seen a woman this tall. Please don't be Mary! Before Mike or I could get a word out she said, "I am checking out, my name is … NO DON'T SAY IT…. "Susan Brooks."

I don't know what came over me (nothing like this had ever happened before,) but I started to laugh and in a split second I knew it was going to be uncontrollable. I wasn't able to get a hold of myself. I bent over the desk, buried my face in my hands, and started to shake with laughter. I shook and shook. My body was straining trying to hold back the laughter. As yet, I have not said one word to this poor woman. I was desperately trying not to laugh in her face. I was in pain and my stomach burned as I tried to maintain control.

Then it happened. For some cruel and unknown reason the entire lobby went dead silent and not one sound was heard. In that very moment, I ripped the loudest fart you ever wanted to hear (it had a nice duration too). It rattled the shades, knocked the clock off the wall, and reverberated down the hallway. Men in the lobby stood with their mouths agape, women grabbed their children, virgins screamed in terror (come to think of it no one screamed).

Well, that was it for me. I couldn't take it any longer. Bent over and red faced (mostly from embarrassment), I stumbled back to my office, fell into my chair, and laughed and laughed.

That poor woman, poor Mikie too, (who had to stay out there) and poor me who had the worst stomach pain I had ever experienced. I stayed in my office until that poor lady checked out. I went back out front. Mike and I had another chuckle. I collected my dollar and went home.

Well, that's it kiddies, hope you had a laugh with me—HUH—WHAT—YES, OK—I guess there is one additional thing. Three weeks later I had to have emergency surgery on an umbilical hernia that I had given myself.

12
HALLUCINATIONS

HALLUCINATIONS

As my Parkinson's has gotten worse, my medications have gotten stronger and the side effects have become more intense. One of the truly unique, interesting, and horrifying side effects is the hallucinations. I never experimented with LSD or other hallucinogens in the 70's, but I have been on a few trips of my own recently. Absolutely the most interesting thing about these hallucinations is that they are so real. I cannot differentiate between reality and a mental fabrication. I would like to tell you about two such instances. "The Women" is the first hallucination I ever experienced and "The Night Visitors" is the most intricate.

THE WOMEN

It was a late summer evening, and I was mowing my lawn on my riding mower. It was near dusk and I was hurriedly trying to complete the job before it got too dark. In the backyard on the north side is "the sewer display." I was coming from the front yard and entered into the back yard when I looked up the hill to the sidewalk and saw two women and a little girl carrying on a conversation. They were wearing bonnets and gray cloaks (very odd attire I thought). I didn't recognize them.

I continued my loop around the house and came into the backyard again, noticing the two women were still carrying on their conversation, but now the little girl was crying. When I got closer to them, the two women looked at me and I gave them a brief wave of acknowledgement. They did not return the wave. Now I became very curious. I made another loop around the house. They were still there, and the little girl was sobbing uncontrollably. I decided to go up and ask them if I could be of any assistance. So I stopped my lawnmower, dismounted, and started walking up the hill. When I got three-quarters of the way up the hill I stopped cold in my tracks: three electrical boxes now occupied the exact spot where the women and the little girl were standing.

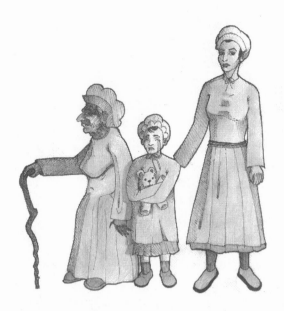

THE NIGHT VISITORS

My sleeping cycle has turned topsy-turvy since I've had Parkinson's. I spend a lot of time dozing off in my power recliner. One of the advantages of this is if I freeze, it usually enables me to get to my feet. I very rarely get a sound night's sleep, as I wake up every 2-½ hours and force myself to go to the bathroom. That's so, if I do wake up frozen and have to go badly, I don't get into trouble.

One night I was lying in my recliner watching TV. It was 2:30 A.M. When I sleep in my recliner I usually sleep in nap-like durations of one to two hours. I was starting to feel a little tired and thought I might try to doze off. As I turned on my side I caught a flash of light in my backyard. I didn't think too much about it as I presumed it was a car passing by. As I gazed out the window I could now see several lights in our yard. I decided to get up and take a look.

I had trouble getting out of the recliner, so I had it power lift me to my feet. I shuffled over to the window, separated two slats in the blinds, and peered out. I was looking at four or five men in my back-yard with flashlights pointed at the ground. They appeared to be look-ing for something, but for the life of me, I couldn't imagine what.

I continued to watch them for a while as they diligently scoured my backyard. As I was standing there, one of them shined a light directly in my eyes. I released the blind instinctively and pulled back. What the hell was going on here? My curiosity quickly changed to fear.

I got down on my hands and knees and crawled through the kitchen and up the stairs to the second level where Kathy was sleeping. I was out of breath, my knees were killing me, but before I awoke Kathy I wanted to make sure that the "night visitors" were still there. So I crawled into the spare bedroom and looked out again. *They were still there all right;* they didn't see me.

I got down on my hands and knees and crawled to our bedroom where I woke Kathy out of a dead sleep. I told her she needed to come with me because there were people in our backyard with flashlights, and I didn't know what was going on. She was groggy but agreed to do so.

She started walking towards our spare bedroom when I told her to get down—I didn't want them to see us. So Kathy got down on her hands and knees, and together we crawled to the bedroom. What a sight that must have been. I told her to look out the window. She did. After several seconds, she turned to me and said, "John, there's nobody out there." It was frightening and impossible for me to comprehend, but indeed, I had hallucinated the entire thing.

13
NO PARKING

NO PARKING

I still drive my car, but some people feel I shouldn't be behind the wheel. After two recent occurrences I may tend to agree with them. I am very defensive about my driving. No, not like being a defensive driver, but being protective about my driving abilities when other people criticize them. Here's my Richard Nixon imitation: "Let me make one thing perfectly clear." No one is a better judge of my driving skills (or lack there of) than myself. I will never put my own well-being or the safety of others at risk because I should not be driving.

Because of my Parkinson's symptoms (rigidity, grip, confusion and drowsiness), I know my skills have diminished, but not to the point that I need to give up driving. There are three complaints that my mom and Kathy have regarding my driving: first, I speed up and slow down; second, I hug the curb; and third, I swerve from side to side. I admit it, I have demonstrated these tendencies, but they are not as bad as they are made out to be.

When I drive with my mom, she hangs her head and refuses to look out the window until the car has come to a stop. She's a nervous wreck the whole way. When we reach our destination I usually make the following announcement: "This is your captain speaking, thank you for choosing Brissette Shuttle Transportation. I hope your trip was an enjoyable one, and I'm sure you are aware your safety is our primary concern. Please do not unbuckle your seat belt or attempt to disembark the vehicle until it has come to a complete stop ... Thank you." She always mumbles something under her breath and gets out.

On the other hand, my wife handles my driving in a different way—she always drives. My mom and my wife also handle another aspect of my driving in a totally different way. My mom doesn't want me to get behind the wheel ever, but if I must and she is around, she insists on going with me. If my wife can't drive she doesn't go.

Three weeks ago I wanted to mow the lawn but discovered I was out of gas. So I opened the door, stuck my head in, and asked Kathy if she wanted to go with me to the gas station. She said no. So I grabbed my keys, the gas can, hopped in the car and drove over to the gas station. It was a beautiful sunny Saturday afternoon. The gas station was very crowded and I was in a hurry because after my chores were done I wanted to play golf.

Just as I pulled into the gas station, someone pulled away from a pump (my lucky day). I accelerated a little and zipped right in. (I was going to be in and out of here in no time.) I stopped the car in front of the pump, opened the door, put the car in reverse, and jumped out. No, it's not a typo, you read it right: I mistakenly put the car in reverse instead of park. As soon as my feet hit the pavement I knew something was wrong, I should have been a rocket scientist. It looked like the car was backing up. MY GOD ... IT WAS BACKING UP!

I immediately jumped back in the car but it was too late. My opened door hit a cement post that protected the pump from nincompoops like me. The door made a terrible groaning sound. I slammed the car into park but not before I bent the door badly. I filled up the gas can and drove over to the side of the lot. The door would open and close but not easily. To close it, you had to slam it hard. To open it you had to use both hands and pull as hard as you could. Well, at least it still worked and it was still attached to the car.

It seems I spend my whole life asking the same question: "What am I going to tell Kathy?" In the words of some great philosopher, Mum's the word. And that's exactly what I did. I just played stupid (not difficult for me). When Kathy asked me about the door a couple days later, I responded, "I dunno, maybe the hinge is loose, I'll check it out." To this day she has never found out. The task now set before me is how to keep Kathy from reading this book.

As I previously stated, my mom does not want me to drive alone. Last week I had to pick up some things at the office supply store. I happened to be visiting my mom and told her I was going over to the store. She had her coat on and was out the door before I could finish the sentence. As usual mom stared at her lap the whole way. We took her car because for some reason I couldn't get the drivers side door open on my car no matter how hard I pulled … Damn cars!

As we drove over to the store my mom asked how long I was going to be. I told her not long at all, I only needed a couple of things. I would be out lickity split. Then an interesting thought came to me: "I wonder how fast I could really make it in and out of the store?"

That little voice spoke to me again ("John, why on earth would you even consider such a thing?) As usual I ignored it. I thought it might be a fascinating little challenge. I told mom to wait in the car. She said OK. I pulled into the parking lot and found a parking spot immediately. I zipped into the spot, hopped out of the car, and started to run into the store.

The scream was unmistakable … it was my name … it was loud … and it was my mother's voice.

JOOOOHHN!!!! HEEEEELLLP!!!!

I wheeled around and saw my mother backing the car out. But why was she screaming for help? Wait a minute—she wasn't backing the car out, she was still in the passenger's seat. Yup, you guessed it: I put the car in reverse again. An invisible driver was driving my mom through the parking lot, backwards. She was still hollering for help and making all sorts of odd noises. People were beginning to look. It was embarrassing.

The car sneaked between two parked cars, just missed running over some poor old lady, jumped the curb, and backed into a telephone pole, and there it came to a stop. My God, my mom was still screaming for me. THIS WAS REALLY EMBARASSING. I walked over to where the car had come to a halt, peered in the open window, and in an irritated and condescending voice asked her why she was screaming so loud. After all, people were looking.

BOY WAS THAT THE WRONG THING TO SAY!

14

LET IT RIDE

LET IT RIDE

It was an overcast and gloomy day, the kind of day you wish you had something neat to do but usually don't. The kind of day you spend your whole morning in the following conversation: you ask your spouse, "What would you like to do today?" She replies, "I don't care, what would you like to do?" To which you respond, "It doesn't matter; what would *YOU* like to do," to which they counter, "I told you it doesn't matter ... anything you want to do is fine with me." And this verbal volley carries on intermittently throughout the rest of the morning.

Several months ago Kathy and I had a similar conversation, except on her third return she asked me if I might like to go to the casino for a little while. I responded with a hearty and excited "You bet" (no pun intended), grabbed my sweater, and got in the car. I didn't check my wallet for money because Kathy never gives me any. (Just joking ... I have to tell you that because she gets real irritated when I say those kinds of things.) Actually, we would probably stop at the bank before we took off, and so we did.

Kathy is not a gambler; she will occasionally play the slot machines but usually she just watches me. I, on the other hand, really enjoy it. I do have two personal rules that I religiously abide by: 1) I never gamble with more money than I can afford to lose (that's why I never take more than $2); and 2) If by chance I should double the amount of money I came with, I put away the original amount for the rest of the time I'm there and only gamble with my winnings. On this day I took $150 out of the bank and we headed up north.

It takes about an hour to get to the casino. It's a very beautiful and pleasant drive along the west side of Michigan. We arrived in no time and pulled into valet parking. I got out, took a deep breath, said a little prayer, and walked through the huge golden doors.

The bells were ringing, the lights were flashing, and you could hear the distinct sound of coins dropping into the metal slot machine hoppers. My heart rate increased and my blood pressure rose. "Ohhh man, I love this."

I like to play several different games: dollar slots, video poker, black jack, but most of all I like a game called "Let It Ride". It is called that because your money rides out of your pocket and into the casino's. This game has a unique entrapment. As you begin each hand you place down three bets and as the game continues you have the option of removing two of them. Thus, it gives the illusion that you could lose more money than you actually do. As a result, you are content with the losses you do have. I am well aware of this mental snare but I play it anyway. I would describe the game for you, but it is totally unimportant to the story, just as this paragraph is.

When I'm in a casino, I am very sensitive about my Parkinson's. I do not want to spill a drink on any of the playing tables. I do not want to freeze at one of the tables. I do not want to shake and drop my cards and I do not want to be caught short and have to shuffle off to a restroom (there are not many and they are hard to find). In short, I do not want to draw any attention to myself, in any way.

We had been at the casino for about 2 ½ hours. We had previously decided that we would leave about 3:00 P.M. It was almost that time now. I still had $65 left so it had been a very nice afternoon. After I left the "let it ride" table and cashed in my chips, we started towards the door. Let it be known that I can never just walk out of a casino. There is always one slot machine or one table that I just have to play before I leave. It's my last chance to hit it big. Don't you *wish* Johnnie Boy?

On this afternoon it was a betting wheel. It's a big wheel with $1, $5, $10, $20, and $50 dollar bills on it. Wherever the wheel stops, if you have placed a bet on that amount, you win your bet times that amount (it isn't necessary that you know this either). I placed a $10 bet on the $20 spot, and one on the $10 spot. That means if I won I would win either $100 or $200. The wheel was spun and after a wrenching 15 seconds or so it landed on the $1 spot. I lost another $20, Kathy grabbed me, and we headed for the door.

As we got within ten feet of the front doors, I had a strong urge to go to the bathroom (#1; for those of you who are detail oriented). I stopped Kathy short of the doors, told her I might have to go to the bathroom soon, and thought it best if I went here. She said she would wait for me here in the lobby, but to please not dilly-dally, as she wanted to get home—and most of all, don't gamble anymore. I told her I wouldn't and hurried off to find the elusive bathroom.

You have to go down several steps to get to the casino floor because it is sunken below the lobby level. Back down in the casino the urge to play just one more time was growing. Unfortunately, the urge to relieve myself was growing ever stronger. It had been ten minutes since I left Kathy. What originally was an occasional glance and lackadaisical search for the public restroom had now become an intense and devoted mission. Why was it so much trouble to find the men's room? Every corner I turned I expected to see my quarry "Gentlemen." In fact, I had been in this corner before. I knew this because of a huge stogie that had been butted out in the urn that I had seen just minutes before. I was starting to feel discomfort. Now, I really had to go. I felt like my bladder was going to burst.

I stood there with my eyes gazing at the urn. I was forced to realize that I was going to commit the unthinkable. NO, *not that!* I was going to ask for directions. I was desperate. I found a houseman and he directed me to the nearest men's room, which wasn't near.

This was not the first time I had been caught short. It has happened several times before. There is one thing that has always remained constant in each instance: The closer you are to your destination, the worse you have to go. As I neared the door, I was sure I wasn't going to make it. I burst through the door, moaning and hanging on for dear life. To my utter amazement the first stall door I pushed on opened and I damn near fell in. I was frantic, I was in distress ... "Help me," I thought. Awkwardly I fumbled for my zipper, lost my grip, and that was it. I stood there and literally filled my shoes. I could not stop. Why did I drink so much? I was sick and humiliated. This couldn't be happening. But yes, it was. I was so embarrassed I almost started crying.

Unfortunately I was wearing light gray jeans. When I looked down I could see a dark five-inch band running down the inside of each leg. I wished I had a cowboy hat and a lariat ... it looked like I was wearing chaps. What in the hell was I going to do now?

The restroom was full. You could hear voices in every direction. I couldn't think of anything to do about my predicament. Then something seemed odd to me. I could hear no one talking. Had everyone left? I opened the door and peered out. Yes indeedy everyone had left. This was my only chance. If I could make it out of the bathroom and into the casino I would be fairly safe. It's dark and everyone is concentrating on the game they are playing. I opened the door and made a mad dash.

The lights were flashing, the bells were ringing, and the sound of coins falling in the hoppers was music to my ears. I made it to the casino floor and no one noticed me. I was right: everyone was concentrating on his or her slot machine. No one paid any attention to me. Even the sound of squishing shoes drew no attention. Yuck!

Now to find Kathy. I knew by now, she was either mad because she thought I was gambling again or worried that something had happened to me. When I saw her I knew in an instant that she was wearing her worried face … PHEW!

"Where have you been?" She demanded. I stepped back and said, "Look." She let out gasp and then followed it up with, "did you pee your pants?" I gave the nod. Now her look changed to concern: "What are we going to do now?"

"Give me a minute and let me think," I said. Then I had a brainstorm. In my case the word "brainstorm" should never be used. It should be substituted with "trouble just waiting to happen." Here was the plan.

I said, "No one is going to notice me as long as I'm in the casino. You go over to valet parking, turn in our ticket, and when our car is brought up to the curb I'll come running up and fall in, smack dab behind you. When I do that, you immediately start walking towards our car. Walk at a little faster pace than normal and I'll follow closely behind you. The only one who will have any chance of seeing me is the valet attendant. You walk right up to the passenger door and at the very last second pull to the right, and go around to the driver's side. I'll slide right in the passenger's door and NO ONE will be the wiser." My brilliance even amazes me sometimes. "Got it? Any questions?"

She just glared at me.

"Are you ready honey?" I asked. She moaned.

There were two driveways. The first one we had to cross was for arriving guests. The second one, for departing guests, is where our car would be brought out. Kathy went over to the valet window and returned.

We only had to wait a few minutes. Here came our car. I hurriedly rushed up the steps and positioned myself behind her. On cue we started to move. We may have looked a little weird, but not real obvious. Our pace was excellent and our goal was straight ahead. We crossed the first drive, and no one was watching us. "God, I am brilliant," I thought to myself.

The attendant got out of our car. He left the drivers side door open and held out his hand. I quickly reminded Kathy to get as close to the car as she could before she moved out of my way. "God I am brilliant." She made her cut and I grabbed the door handle and started to get in. "HEY BUDDY, WHAT ARE YOU DOING? THAT'S MY CAR."—*W h a t*? *I couldn't believe it … This wasn't our car.*

I stood there, aghast, with my jaw dropped open. I watched this stranger hand the valet attendant a buck, slide down into the driver's seat, and pull away.

There I stood, alone, in front of the whole damn casino and everyone was watching.

Out of nowhere a loud voice from behind me bellowed, "LOOK THAT GUY PEED HIS PANTS!" I turned to see who said that, and my eyes bulged in total disbelief: I was standing smack dab in front of a bus filled with college kids.

Why do these things always happen to me?

15

THE HANDYMAN

THE HANDYMAN

A MULTITUDE OF PROBLEMS

The Parkinson's patient never knows what to expect from one day to the next. The symptoms never go away but they vary in intensity from day to day. When you add the side effects of the medications, any given day can be a major challenge. Will my hands work today, will I be able to walk, will I be able to get over the hump (but not too far over) will I be able to function at all? Facing this everyday can be frightening and frustrating, but it can also create some hilarious situations.

Two years ago my sister Barbara and my brother-in-law Dave bought a beautiful previously owned home. I had recently retired and was beginning to get bored without much to do. One day when my sister happened to mention to me that she was going to hire a painter to paint her living room, a plumber to do some work in her bath, and a yardman to do some landscaping, I stepped forward and in a self-assuring tone said, "Barb, don't do that. I can do all those things for you and it won't cost you dime. What do you say?"

Well, I could read her "not on your life" facial expression very well but chose to ignore it. After a moment of silence, the words I wanted to hear rolled off her lips. "I guess so … that would be great".

When I told Kathy my plan, she just shook her head and said "John, are you sure you know what you are getting yourself into? When a job goes *well* for you around our house it usually requires three to four trips to the hardware store, it costs us twice as much as it should have, and you usually get so angry and frustrated that I have to stay away from you the rest of the day.

To which I replied in a condescending voice, "I won't have any problems, don't worry about that." As I heard her mumble, "famous last words," I thought to myself, "Women just don't understand."

This was going to be great. Dave and Barb both worked, which meant I would have the entire house to myself. I would be able to work uninterrupted, complete the job, and return home in no time. After Barb explained to me what she wanted done, I carefully calculated the time involved and figured I would be done in three to four days—max.

On Sunday morning I packed up the tools I would need, stuffed a few extra clothes into my duffle bag, kissed Kathy goodbye, and headed out the door. As I got into the car, Kathy hollered out in a pleading voice, "Are you really sure you know what you are getting yourself into?" "Pessimist," I thought, started the car, waved good-bye, and away I went.

When I got to my sister's house I surveyed the situation. I decided that as long as the weather forecast for Monday was good I would begin outside in the yard. There were two things Barb wanted completed. The lawn needed edging badly as it had grown about four inches over the sidewalk and driveway, and in the back yard by the family room ivy had gone wild and was growing everywhere and she wanted it all removed.

I decided I would start with the edging; it was the easiest of the jobs and I wanted to make sure that I accomplished as much as possible the first day to put my sister's mind at ease. When I saw how desperately their lawn needed edging I was glad I had brought my edger from home. It was electric, but a heavy-duty model and would chew through the sod lickity split.

It was 9:10 A.M. I plugged in my extension cord, plugged in the edger, squeezed the trigger, and started to push. But I wasn't moving; what the hell? Nothing was moving. I squeezed the trigger several times but still nothing happened. I checked and double-checked the connections, everything was intact … I figured I must have blown a breaker.

I went looking for the breaker box. In the garage: nothing. Down in the basement: nothing. Back in the new family room: nothing. I did find a breaker box there but it was only for the electric starter on a gas space heater. I searched and searched but I could not locate it. The last thing I wanted to do was call Barb or Dave. I was getting very irritated. It was now 10:20 A.M and I hadn't accomplished one damn thing.

***Bingo* …** What an idiot, why didn't I think of that before?—The box should be somewhere in the basement. All I had to do was follow the wires to the breaker box. That's what I did, and sure enough, I found it hidden behind the furnace. What numbskull would do that? Well, I didn't want to waste any time dwelling on that, so I quickly opened the cover. To my dismay, not one breaker appeared to be tripped. How could that be?

I stood there dumb-founded staring at the breaker panel. I finally surmised that maybe it was a bad breaker or it had tripped just a little, not enough to tell. In addition to being unable to determine if any breaker had been tripped, I couldn't identify which breaker I was supposed to be looking for; half the breakers had no explanation on them and the other half you couldn't read. I said to myself, "John, before you leave Thursday (I had just eliminated the three day option and was now sure it would take at least four days to finish) you are going to re-label this box."

I'm sure the problem wasn't my edger; it had to be a breaker. The only reasonable solution was to reset all the breakers—yes that would do it. I smugly said out loud, "There's more than one way to skin a cat." (Where did that saying ever come from, anyway? Why would anyone want to skin a cat?) So I repeatedly switched every breaker off and on. Well, that's that I said out loud. I put a confident grin on my face and raced up stairs. *I had to get going.*

When I opened the door one would have thought it was Christmas Eve. There where red and white lights, numbers and words flashing everywhere. Oh my God ... I had restarted every electrical appliance in the house. What the hell was I going to do now? There was no way to avoid it, when Barb and Dave got home, I was going to have to tell them what happened. Alarm clocks had to be reset, answering machines would have to be re-programmed and so on. The only thing I could do now was reset as many as I could and leave the rest until my sis got home. She was going to kill me.

I headed outside and then I felt it. My toes started to stiffen a little. My fingers in my left hand started to stiffen too, and when I took a step forward I was unable to move my foot with ease. In all the commotion I had forgotten to take my medicine. I only had a few seconds before I would be in real trouble. I raced into the house as best I could and sat on a kitchen chair. I made it. My pills were at hand. I swallowed my regular dose and one more pill.

There I sat for the next 20 minutes unable to move freely. I was wasting valuable time.

Finally, I felt my body start to relax and come back to me. The tremors and stiffness were starting to subside. At last I could finally start edging the lawn. It was now 1:35 P.M. It had been over 4 ½ hours since I started this morning and I hadn't cut so much as six inches of the lawn. Damn ... Barb and Dave would be home in less than 3 ½ hours. I had to move fast.

I went back outside. At least I was sure of one thing: I had fixed the problem.

I grabbed the edger, lined it up along the driveway, pulled the trigger, and pushed forward. Nothing happened. "Damn it, what is going on here, I don't believe this. Why am I being tortured?" I was ready to smash my edger into a million pieces. "Get a hold of yourself." I was starting to flake out big time. I ran downstairs to check the breaker box, and again I found nothing. What was I going to do? I knew one thing I wasn't going to do—reset all the breakers.

I started to think that maybe Kathy was right; maybe I was in over my head. I sat there for fifteen minutes trying to figure out what was going on and what I had to do next. Finally it came to me: maybe the problem was with the outlet. As I headed upstairs I saw Barb's electric broom standing in the corner. I grabbed it and brought it along. I plugged it into the same outlet that my edger was plugged into. "Please don't let it work," I thought to myself. I turned on the electric broom and it purred away.

That left only one possibility. The problem had to be with my edger. It was 3:05 P.M. The clock was my enemy and still ticking away. Barb should be home in an hour and half and I hadn't even turned my edger on yet. This was definitely not going the way I had planned.

"Ok, *John*, you bubblehead ... you never should have offered to help." Then that other little man in my head started to talk to me (you know, the one who goads you on to do something you know you shouldn't), "Stop it John, are you some kind of weasel? You aren't going to sit there and let a few little setbacks prevent you from completing your task? Get a grip mama's boy, you still have time left to get something done. Fix your edger and get going."

"Ok, I will," I said reluctantly to myself. I went into the house, got a couple of screwdrivers, and took the cover off my edger handle. Immediately, two springs came flying out. "Oh God, I wish I had a gun!!" I looked inside the handle, but I couldn't see anything that looked wrong, but I knew two things were definitely wrong: the edger didn't work (you're a genius) and I had no idea where those two springs went.

I said, "Before you do anything else stupid, *think*". The words of my Dad came back to me, "John, use your head. Stop and think before you go off half-cocked—just think." He even bought me a large sign for my room that just had the word "Think" on it. So I did. I checked all the connections: the problem was not with the extension cords. The problem wasn't with the breakers: I had reset every one of them. The problem wasn't with the outlet: I plugged in the electric broom and it worked fine. The problem had to be with my edger and it most likely was the switch.

I called every hardware store within a five-mile radius but no one sold a replacement switch. That left only one other option. I would have to buy a new edger. That would probably run about $59. As I sat there confused and feeling beaten, I mumbled to myself, "That's great, you've spent the entire day doing nothing, and now it's going to cost you $59."

Well, I couldn't waste any more time. I went inside and changed my clothes. I put on a brand new pair of Dockers I had just bought, a clean shirt, grabbed my wallet and keys, swallowed a few pills, and drove over to the nearest builder's store. I located the edgers. I was aghast. The cheapest edger they had, the same model as mine, was now $89.

How in the hell do I get myself into these things? I grabbed the new edger, which was in a very large box, and headed to the cashier.

I took about twenty steps when, unexpectedly, the lower half of my body froze but the upper half did not. The result was, I rocketed forward at lightning speed, faster than a speeding bullet, shuffling my feet a few inches at a time on my tiptoes. I looked like Rudolf Nuriev running a hundred yard dash. It was a sight to see. As I raced down the main aisle, I passed an elderly couple who had a look of horror on their faces. They could tell as well as I could that I was going to lose it. With a large box in my arms and nothing to protect myself I lunged forward and slid into third base, face first ... SAFE!

People came running from all directions and surrounded me. I could hear their voices: "Are You OK?" "Don't move, you may have broken something"; "I think he's drunk"—no, I think someone was chasing him"; "He's too old to be running." I was embarrassed and just wanted to get the hell out of there, fast.

My knees were killing me. I had landed on them, tore both legs in my Dockers and both knees were badly scraped and bleeding. The first words out of my mouth were, *"I'm alright! I just want to get up!"*

I quickly got to my feet (I wasn't frozen anymore and found I was able to walk normally). I grabbed my box and went to the cashier. My knees were killing me. I couldn't help noticing the stares as I walked through the parking lot. When I got to my sister's house I had no time to change. Someone would be home any minute, and I had to get something done. I quickly assembled the edger, plugged it in, and started to edge, but nothing happened. I stood there with my mouth dropped open, torn pants, and bloody knees. This can't be happening. I was sitting on the front porch when Dave pulled in and drove into the garage. I heard him go into the house and set some packages on the kitchen table. He came to the front door.

"How's it going, Johnson? Did you have good day?"

"Well let me tell you Dave, I've had an absolute terrible day." I stood up and turned around.

"What in the hell happened to you?" he gasped. "Are you alright?"

"Yes," I replied. "I'm okay but I'm about ready to pack up and go home, or blow my brains out, which ever is easier."

"Well, that doesn't sound very good John. Let me go in and change, grab a couple of cold ones, and I'll be right back out." Okay.

"Okay," I said.

While Dave was changing I went in, washed off my knees, sprayed some antiseptic on them, and changed my pants. So much for my brand new Dockers. I was now $130 in the hole.

I went back outside, grabbed the new edger again, and pulled the trigger. Nothing happened. Get *me* a pistol right now I want to end this … I do! "I CAN'T TAKE THIS ANY LONGER!" I screamed out loud. I felt like running up and down the street naked with ax in my hand screaming, "The bats are coming, the bats are coming!" I know, it doesn't make sense to me either, but who can explain insanity? *Please,* take me to the booby hatch … the damn edger still didn't start. Honestly I thought I was losing my mind. I felt like crying. I had just wasted the entire day accomplishing absolutely nothing. "Why do these things happen to me?" I pleaded.

Dave came out the front door with two cold beers in his hand and handed me one. I took a long gulp. Boy, did that taste good. I lit up a cigar and started to calm down a little. Dave said, "Now tell me what happened today." I told him the whole miserable scenario. "Oh man," he sighed and started to laugh.

"What's so funny?" I asked a little perturbed. "John, did you happen to notice that the outlet you were using has a GFI on it? (For those of you who don't know what a GFI is, it's a Ground Fault Interrupter, an outlet with its own tiny circuit breaker.) I'm sure that's your problem. It just has to be reset."

"No, I didn't notice, Dave, or I would have reset it. You usually only see them in bathrooms or kitchens," I replied. Dave said, "I'll check it now."

He got up, pushed the reset button on the outlet, took the edger, and pulled the trigger. It started right up. "I can't figure it out! I plugged Barb's electric broom into the same outlet and it worked just fine, but it shouldn't have."

"How could that be?"

"I'll tell you how," Dave said with a bit of laughter in his voice. "Barb's electric broom also operates on batteries. So when you plugged in the broom and there was no power the batteries took over." I picked up my stuff, put it in the garage, told Dave I was done for the day, and went into the house.

When Barb came home I heard the two of them splitting a gut in the kitchen at my expense. But that's OK; because it really was kind of funny. At dinner we had another good laugh about the day's events. I only hoped tomorrow would be better; it couldn't be any worse, or *so I thought!*

I rose early the next morning. I had a lot of catching up to do and I wanted to get going. I wasn't in the mood to do any edging today, and besides it looked like it might rain, so I decided to work in the bathroom.

Barbara said the shower would not maintain a comfortable temperature. She wanted to hire a plumber to do the job; but that wasn't really necessary as it was a very simple repair. All I had to do was shut off the hot and cold water in the basement (I couldn't shut it off in the bathroom because they didn't have individual shut-offs for the tub), and install a new shower cartridge. That was that ... finished.

I went to the basement, shut off the hot and cold water, and went back upstairs to the bathroom. "This was going to be a much better day than yesterday", I said confidently to myself.

The tub valve was a single handle type. I unscrewed the knob, took off the face plate, and removed the mixing cartridge. The cartridge must have been on there a very long time because it was extremely difficult to remove, but I finally got it off with vice grips and a little sweat. Everything was going along very nicely—too nicely.

This was going to be a great day!

I installed the new mixing cartridge, replaced the nut that held it in place (I could reinstall the cover plate and knob later after I checked for leaks), and headed downstairs to turn the water back on. I opened both valves and ran like hell upstairs to make sure there weren't any leaks. I knew this was going to be a great day. I didn't see any leaks but I wanted to give it about an hour or so just to make sure.

Finally, something was going right. It was only 11:35 A.M. and I had already finished the plumbing. "Bring on the next task," I smugly said to myself. It was still gloomy outside so I thought I would paint the living room next. I went to the basement, got the paint, my brushes and roller, and the rest of the tools and supplies I would need. However, I did forget drop cloths. I wasn't too concerned because I'm a very good painter and rarely make any kind of a mess. The only thing I was a little concerned about was that this was brand new carpeting and it was very expensive. "No problem," I told myself, "just be extra careful."

I set up my ladder, popped the top off the paint can, stirred it for a minute, and started to place it on the shelf of the ladder. That little voice spoke to me again. "John, don't do that, you might spill it; at least find some kind of drop cloth." I'll be very, very careful, I convinced myself, and set the can on the shelf. I bent down to pick up my paint brush and lost my balance.

Instinctively, I reached to grab something to save myself, but before my brain clicked in my hand found the ladder, and the full can of paint went flying. I watched it (in what appeared to be slow motion) turn one and a half revolutions and land upside down with a dull THWAP on the floor. "OH MY GOD!" I screamed, as I went flying backwards across the room, arms flailing, smashing into the wall, and leaving a large dent in the drywall.

"NO, NO, NO," I screamed even louder. "NO, NO." That's all that came out of mouth. I kept screaming over and over again.

I crawled across the floor, righted the paint can, and with both hands cupped, began scooping mauve paint back into the can. I scooped and scooped and then I heard the most unusual sound come from upstairs. It actually sounded like someone had fired a gun. "What the hell was that," I yelled as mauve paint kept spreading wider. Why didn't I listen to Kathy?

Then I saw it. I couldn't believe my eyes. Please ... this couldn't be. Then that little voice spoke to me again: "That's right, Johnny boy, you may think you are having another hallucination but you are not. There really is water coming out of the ceiling." I watched the small water spot grow bigger and bigger. What in the hell was that sound, and what was on going upstairs?

I wiped my hands on my shirt and pants and raced upstairs. I stood in the doorway of the bathroom in total disbelief. There was a gush of water pouring out of the handle area of the tub. It looked like it was coming from a fire hose. Ninety percent of the water was in the tub. The other ten percent was splashing onto the floor and seeping down to the living room ceiling. I quickly grabbed my pliers from the floor and ran over to the tub to turn the valve off. To my utter surprise, there was no cartridge.

Ring-a-ding-ding. I knew what the gunshot was. The water pressure was so strong it blew the valve right out of the pipe.

"Don't just stand there ... do something, knucklehead!"

I was running so fast down the steps that for a moment I thought I might actually be able to fly. I reached the shutoffs in an Olympic record setting 4.1 seconds and closed them. I ran upstairs like a madman, three stairs at a time, and went back to the living room.

I dropped to my knees and continued to scoop up paint. The spot had grown to over four feet. What in the hell was I going to do now? After several more handfuls, I had scooped up as much residual paint as

I could. I looked up at the ceiling. The spot was now over a foot wide and still dripping. As I sat there, my eyes were diverted to the dent in the wall. How was I ever going to fix that? I felt sick to my stomach. I was mildly shaking (not from Parkinson's) and had to admit to myself that maybe, just maybe, I had gotten myself in over my head. It was time to think again. What did I need to do first?

The dent in the wall was the least of my concerns. The water was off so my immediate attention was directed towards the spilled paint. I knew what I had to do: get the stain out of the carpet (I should be a MENSA candidate). And so I began. I went to the garage and got Dave's shop vac. I went to the laundry room and got a pail that I filled with cold water. "Oh god, I hope I am doing the right thing," I thought. I poured the entire 1-½ gallons of water on to the spot and began to frantically suck it up with the shop vac. Two things were in my favor: it was a very expensive carpet, which meant it was durable and would resist stains, and it was latex paint (which meant it was water soluble). I repeated these steps six or seven times. Each time it looked a little better. After about an hour I thought I should probably go up and check the leak in the bathroom.

The dripping had stopped. The spot was about two feet in diameter. I found the cartridge and discovered that during the process of removing the old cartridge I had stripped the threads in the valve, which caused the problem. This meant that I had to go to the hardware store and buy a new valve and cartridge. Before I left, I grabbed four or five towels and laid them over the paint spill and did a very poor calypso dance on top of them. I hurried off to the hardware.

It was now 2:30 in the afternoon. I purchased a new valve and cartridge, a five-gallon pail of joint compound for the dent in the wall, a new gallon of paint, and a quart of spackling for the ceiling. The total cost was $67.19; I was now $197.19 in the hole and hadn't completed one repair in the house. I also figured that it would take six days to complete the jobs.

I arrived back at Barb's house, went in to the living room, picked up the towels, and threw them into the washing machine. For the first time during this whole fiasco I felt like I might actually be able to get the spot removed. Another four gallons of water and forty-five minutes later I had accomplished my task. I honestly could not tell where the stain had been. The carpet was still very wet, however, I would deal with that problem later. I said a silent prayer that no one would come into this room in their stocking feet.

Here came that little man again. "Well fat-head, what are you going to tell Barb and Dave you did all day? They will be home soon, and again you have accomplished nothing." "I'll think of something," I said, and went upstairs to the bathroom. An hour and fifteen minutes later I finally accomplished something. The valve and the cartridge were replaced. There appeared to be no leaks.

Now let me tell you, my nerves were shot, I had a splitting head-ache, and I felt defeated. I started to laugh. It really was funny. In fact it was hilarious. How could one person have so many things go wrong? It was beyond belief. I continued to laugh until my stomach ached. I started feeling better. Laughing always makes one feel better. Now, I needed to think.

Barb or Dave should be home very soon. I couldn't tell them I had another disastrous day, could I? No I couldn't. So I had to think of something fast!

After a few minutes it came to me in a revelation. I raced over to the hardware store and bought a large roll of black plastic sheeting (another $9.62 wasted and the combined total was now $206.81). I hurried back to the house and cut the plastic into large sections and taped them to the side walls. It hid the dent quite nicely.

With that disguise in place I ran up to the bathroom, snatched Barb's hair dryer, and began drying the water spot in the living room. It was now 5:07 P.M. I realized I only had minutes left before someone came home.

After several minutes the ceiling appeared to be pretty dry. If you looked really hard and knew what to look for you could see a faint water stain, but I hoped the casual observer wouldn't notice.

I scurried upstairs to the bathroom—(there were absolutely no leaks, praise the Lord)—reattached the faceplate, the handle knob, and cleaned up the mess as I heard Barbara's car pull into the garage. "Get set John, in just a few minutes you will have the opportunity to take the final oral examination for an honorary membership into the liars club."

"Well, how did it go today? Better than yesterday I hope," were the first words out of Barb's mouth.

The little man said, "Spew them lies, Johnny Boy, spew them lies."

"Pretty good. I didn't get as much completed as I wanted to. I kind of had a bad Parkinson's day (sometimes my disease can come in real handy), but I did complete your tub repair, and got the living room all covered up to begin painting in the morning."

"Well that's not too bad I guess," she replied, "but at this rate you are going to be here a month" she snickered. Ouch, that hurt. At dinner, Dave questioned me, "Why do you have plastic on the walls if you are going to paint them?" I replied that I did not want to get splatters on the wall as they are too hard to remove and show badly when you paint over them.

The rest of the evening I was on needles and pins and prayed no one would go into the living room without shoes on or peek under the plastic. As my head hit my pillow I said a silent, "Thank you."

I rose early again the next morning. I met Barb in the kitchen and she asked me, "What do you have planned for today, John?"

I wanted to tell her that I felt like blowing up her house with me in it … but I really couldn't do that—I didn't have any dynamite. With that option eliminated I told her I planned on painting the living room and finishing the edging. Barb went off to work and I went into the living room to check the carpet.

It was still pretty damp but you couldn't see any stain. Thank God!

Before I started painting again I had a mission to accomplish. I scoured the garage, the attic, and the basement, but could not find a single fan.

I grabbed my keys and drove over to the hardware store. They were beginning to say hi to me on a first name basis. I bought a fan for $14.11, bringing my total to $220.92. Kathy was going to kill me when she found out how much money I had spent, and I was quite sure this wasn't the last of it either.

When I got back to the house I took the plastic off the walls and laid it on the floor. Then I started the fan to help dry out the damp carpet and began to paint. I completed the first coat in about three hours. It looked really good but it did need another coat. Now I had to address the dent in the wall.

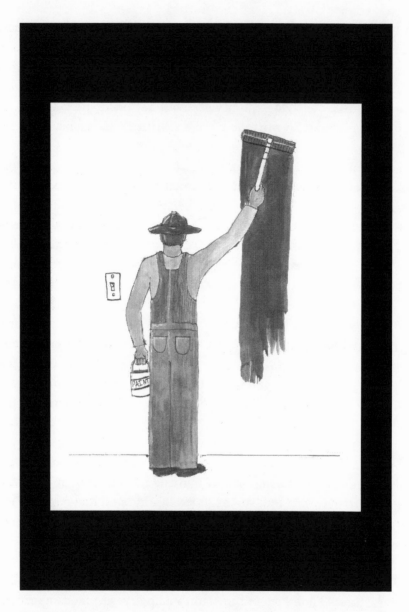

Short of replacing a whole section of drywall I felt I could fill in the dent with joint compound and nobody should be able to tell. I got some sandpaper and roughed up the area where the dent was. I slopped on some joint compound and smoothed it out. This procedure usually required three applications with vigorous sanding in between. It could be a very nasty job but what choice did I have? None. A plus of using joint compound is that it dries very rapidly. By the end of the day, I should be able to have all three applications done and one coat of paint, too. But first I wanted to repair and paint the water spot on the ceiling.

I was reasonably surprised that the ceiling looked as good as it did. But it really should be patched. I took out my chisel and began chipping the damaged plaster. When I was done I had chipped out a two-foot circle about a ½ inch deep. I opted for spackling for the ceiling because it is a more durable product. I applied my first coat and went back to my painting.

It was now 3:20 in the afternoon. All I had left to do was sand down my last coat of joint compound and spackling and put on a primer and one coat of paint. The other three walls were all done. It was still a couple of hours before Dave or Barb got home. I had plenty of time. I had stayed at my tasks all day and had worked very hard. I thought I would take a little break.

I had kept up on my medicine very well. I was a little more over the hump than I wanted to be, but I couldn't take a chance of freezing and wasting any valuable time. I went to the kitchen and grabbed myself a cold one. They sure can taste good when you are tired. I sat down in Dave's easy chair and turned on CNN for just a minute.

"OH MY GOD, WHAT HAPPENED? WHAT HAVE YOU DONE?" I bolted out of the easy chair, dumped my beer on the carpet, and stood red faced and unable to speak. I watched my sister as she visually inspected the patched wall and ceiling. I had fallen sound asleep and it was now 5:30 P.M.

"Barb," I said frantically, "It looks worse than it really is. Trust me."

"You boob," she replied. "What happened?" I spit out the whole story. "The only thing I can say is you're lucky. Dave called and said he wouldn't be home until after 8:00 P.M. as he had a business dinner to attend. You had better get everything fixed by then. What can I do to help?" "Well, really nothing Barb, if Dave won't be home until 8:00 P.M. I'll be OK, I promise."

As she turned to leave and go upstairs, I saw her roll her eyes and heard her mumble something about her brother. I was pretty sure it wasn't very complimentary.

At 7:50 P.M. I finished all the repairs in the living room, painted the wall, and had everything cleaned up and put away. When Barb came back downstairs she said, "After Dave goes to sleep tonight I'm going to come down and have a talk with you, OK." I said Ok but I wasn't looking forward to it.

At 11:15 P.M. she came into the family room and sat down. "John, why don't you quit, go back home, and let me hire someone to finish the work. I don't want to see you hurt yourself, you might never leave." We both let out a chuckle.

"Barb, I don't want to do that," I replied. "I told you I was going to do these repairs for you and I have every intention of completing the job. I've had a few misfortunes. They could have happened to anybody."

"Maybe John" she responded, "but they always seem to happen to you. Are you sure?"

"Yes I am," I answered, mildly irritated. "OK," she said. "If you change your mind let me know." And she went up to bed.

Morning came fast. I slept in a little later than normal. As I lay in bed I asked myself, "Why do these things always happen to me." That little man in my head jumped right up and spoke his mind. "Listen here, Johnny boy, I'll tell you why. You are an idiot. That's why. You don't know when to say no. You are stubborn and you don't think …" "GET LOST," I said, and got out of bed.

I told myself that this day was going to be different! I was going to do everything in my power to see that nothing went wrong today. I was determined.

I took a shower, got dressed, and headed out the door. I stopped in my tracks. It was pouring outside. What was I going to do now? Nothing, bubblehead. The only jobs I had to do were outside. My luck. Damn, I could be here a week. What was I going to tell Kathy? I sat around all day, watched TV, and napped.

It finally stopped raining in the evening. The forecast for the next day was clearing skies. That was fantastic news, because hopefully I could complete my work. I missed Kathy very much and I wanted to go home.

The skies in the morning were cloudy and gray but it wasn't raining. Hallelujah!

Reluctantly I took my new edger out of the garage, connected the extension cord, plugged it in, and pulled the trigger. It made the most wonderful whirring sound. I placed it on the edge of the driveway and pushed. It didn't push easily; the sod was very thick. This was a much harder job than I had expected, but I was determined. I was going to get it done.

Four and a half hours later I was finished. I swept up the sidewalk and the driveway. Now I had just one job left to do. I grabbed some work gloves and a trash can and went into the back yard to pull out the ivy. I was dead tired. Every bone in my body ached. I couldn't think of any time I worked harder. It was 1:15 P.M. I didn't want to rest for fear of falling asleep again. I was so sore I didn't want to stiffen up and not be able to resume working.

Barb was right; the ivy was very thick and was growing out of control. It all needed to be removed. I got down on my hands and knees and began pulling it out. This was also more difficult than I had imagined. I worked at it for about thirty minutes and determined that I couldn't do this much longer. It was just too hard for me and I felt I was getting nowhere. Some of the vines were very thick and securely attached to ground and the house. I could not pull these vines out.

'What am I going to do?" I said to myself. "There's got be some other way."

"If I only had something to—yes, that's it, that's my solution." I'll get Dave's hedge trimmers and I'll cut right through that ivy like a hot knife through butter."

I got the hedge trimmer and my extension cord, turned it on, and started making wide sweeping motions through the ivy. This really is *working* well. It was cutting through the ivy very quickly.

I had cut through most of the ivy on the ground and was nearing the base of the house. "That was a funny sound," I thought. Then I heard another odd sound, but I couldn't quite make it out with the hedge trimmers still running, so I shut them off. I still couldn't place that sound.

"There aren't any rattle snakes around here. What is that sound?" I questioned myself, again. Then I smelled it. Rotten eggs. "OOOO-HHH NNOOO, it's natural gas!" "I cut a gas line. But what gas line?" I thought. "What difference does that matter you jerk, a gas line is a gas line and that hissing sound means the gas is escaping very fast," the little voice said to me.

I felt like puking. I hadn't had a single day when something serious didn't go wrong. I couldn't take any more of this. I suddenly wondered if death by natural gas asphyxiation was painless and quick. I was tempted to find out but I didn't have the time. I had to get the leak stopped temporarily.

I ran to the basement and snatched a roll of duct tape (the handyman's favorite tool) and raced back outside. I found the cut gas line and started to wrap duct tape around it until the hissing sound stopped. I went inside and called the gas company and notified them of the gas leak. They were there in just minutes. The repairman shut off the gas and informed me that if I wanted him to repair the gas line it would cost $103.56, or I could call a licensed plumber to fix it.

I explained my predicament to him. I didn't have time to call anyone else, so I asked him if he could repair it now. He said yes and went to his truck to get his tools. When he returned I paid $103.56, which made a grand total of out of pocket losses $320.48. How did I ever let this happen? I asked the repairman if he would please hurry because my sister or brother-in-law would be home soon. He said he understood, and would go as fast as he could.

I looked down the driveway and couldn't believe my eyes. Walking up the drive was Kathy. I was so glad to see her; I missed her so much! But I knew I was never going to hear the end of this.

"Oh God, how do I get myself into these things?"

16
EUREKA

EUREKA

"Eureka." The word means, "I found it." Thank God it didn't take me my whole life to find it. With many people it does, and there are others who never find it at all. I feel very sad for those who never realize the powers they have.

What I have found is how to enjoy my life, regardless of what hurdles are placed in my way. Life is too short and too precious to waste one moment because that moment will never be available again. It is gone forever ... history.

If I could have planned and written my life story, there are definite chapters that I would have omitted, and Parkinson's disease would head up the list. However, neither I nor anyone else has that divine capability, so I will make the best of what I have. We must face life's challenges head on. Acknowledge them and overcome them. Do not let depression overtake you, and believe me, you do have the internal strength to do this. Nobody said life was going to be easy, at least nobody said it to me.

In order for us to truly enjoy our life there are several key elements that must exist.

Family and friends. We are social animals by nature. We do not function well when we are alone. When tragedy hits us we need the love and compassion of others to help us through the tough times. It is unfathomable for me to imagine handling my Parkinson's alone. Regardless of what miseries I may face, I will not face them alone and therefore those tragedies will never beat me.

The paths we choose. What we put into our lives is exactly what we get out of it. The paths we choose to follow and the decisions we choose to make are our choices alone. An upbeat and optimistic attitude will reap positive results. A regretful and angry attitude will reap negative results. You can bet on it.

Patch ill feelings. I have witnessed many people who exist in dysfunctional families of one form or another. Please heed my advice. Put any petty differences aside (and trust me they are petty) and put to rest any ill feelings you may have. Say, "I'm sorry" regardless of who may be at fault. Underneath all the bitterness there is still a foundation of love. Someday you may realize all too late what a horrible mistake you have made and all the precious moments you have lost can never be recaptured again. That will be a part of your life that will be gone forever.

Say, "I love you" to those who are dear to you regardless of whom they are: man or woman, child or adult. Just do it. It may be difficult at first but mark my words, in time it will become much easier and you will find a most wonderful transformation has taken place. Before long your loved ones will be saying, "I love you," in return. At that point your life will take on a whole new meaning.

There are no guarantees in life; there is no rose garden. Life can be cruel and dish out some very difficult obstacles to face. It's imperative that we control or remedy those that we can. It is even more important that we *accept* the others as bad breaks, and discover ways of dealing with them, thus making our life easier and more enjoyable. Wasting precious time trying to understand why bad things happen to us gets us nowhere. Eventually it will direct us to a path of self-pity and depression. Choose the other path.

When I was first diagnosed with Parkinson's disease I was convinced that I could not do the things I used to do. My life as I knew it would be changed forever. But "O ye of little faith." I found out later that nothing could be further from the truth. All I had to do was find alternate ways of accomplishing the things I loved to do. I found that I could climb the steps in the stands at the football stadium, I could carry a tray in a restaurant without spilling, I could drive the car, and I could speak in public. All of these things, along with others, I thought would be beyond my limited abilities, but through want and desire and the help of my loved ones—EUREKA, I found the way.

Whoever said laughter is the best medicine was a genius. It is our shield against pity and depression. When we laugh at ourselves, or in the face of misfortune, we have disarmed our enemy. Most adversities have a funny side to them if only we choose to look for it. It feels good to laugh. A smile can make your whole day enjoyable. It's infectious.

Just the mere fact that you wake up in the morning should put an instant smile on your face ... I know it does me! Change your life now. Try this every morning when you wake up; throw back your covers, get out of bed as fast as you can, and in an excited voice (pumping your fists, putting your hands over your head, or doing whatever it takes to get yourself geared up) scream as loudly as you can "THIS IS GOING TO BE A GREAT DAY!" and mean it. After you peel your spouse off the ceiling or they get finished dialing the insane asylum, you will find that this upbeat attitude will influence your whole day. Try it—it really works.

Make the best of every situation that you are confronted with. I do realize that every situation may not have a funny side to it, like the loss of a child. Some crises are so devastating that they are almost unbearable. However, there is a time for sorrow and mourning but more importantly there is a time of acceptance and getting on with your life. There is little time to be sad but a lot of time to be happy. I love the old adage, "laugh and the world laughs with you; cry and you cry alone." It's so true.

Lastly, enjoy your life, whatever the circumstances may be. Laugh in the face of misfortune, laugh in the face of depression, and laugh in the face of self-pity—just laugh. Tomorrow I want you to be able to say, **"EUREKA."**

About the Author

I was an average kid, born into an average family, raised in an average neighborhood. However, one thing that wasn't average—our family was never embarrassed to say "I love you". It was as easy as saying hello.

I grew up in Royal Oak, Michigan, and attended Dondero High School, where my outlook on life began to broaden and I discovered humor as a means of communication. In college, at Michigan State University, my examination of the world and appreciation for life began to manifest itself. As I matured I developed an understanding on how precious life was and how vital it was to have family and friends. Through all these years I never lost the ability to see the humorous side of anything.

My career path led me to the hospitality industry where I managed several hotels and restaurants. I have always been a hard-worker and believe that you are not owed anything. What you accomplish or achieve in your life is based solely on the efforts that you put forth. That is one value I will always carry with me.

At age 45 I was devastated when I was diagnosed with Parkinson's disease. But I never let depression, anger, or self-pity take over my life. I accepted my condition for what it was and moved forward to make the best of what I had.

I currently live in Rockford, Michigan with my wife Kathy and have two children Jason and Beth and a twelve-year old wonder dog named Tyler (a golden retriever).

I have developed a fresh and positive attitude. As a result I have found peace, love, and purpose in my life. The joy of living has returned to me. I have rediscovered the exhilaration that humor can have in my life and that has become my focus.

978-0-595-42500-6
0-595-42500-3

Made in the USA
Lexington, KY
27 March 2011